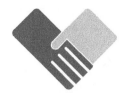

INTENTIONAL CAREGIVING

TEN PRINCIPLES
on How *to* Become *an*
Exceptional CNA

CHRISTINA MILES

THE INSIGHTFUL EDITOR

First Edition, January 2021.

THE INSIGHTFUL EDITOR

Linda Ruggeri
theinsightfuleditor.com
linda@theinsightfuleditor.com

Published by The Insightful Editor (Linda Ruggeri) theinsightfuleditor.com

Proofreading by Marcella Lopez, marcellahealthcare.com
Cover & Interior Design by Melinda Martin Publishing Services

ISBN-10: 0-9992780-9-3
ISBN-13: 978-0-9992780-9-3

Intentional Caregiving: Ten Principles on How to Become an Exceptional CNA is available at quantity discounts for bulk purchases for educational, business, sales, or promotional use. For information, please contact caregiveracademy1@gmail.com.

*This book is dedicated to
all the people who lost their lives to COVID-19,
and to their loved ones*

And to my beloved grandparents, Grace and Jerry Beard

CONTENTS

INTRODUCTION

Hi, I'm Christina Miles ("Nina") and this book will give you the tools you need to have a successful career as a Certified Nursing Assistant (CNA).

Ever since I was a little girl, I've always wanted to write a book. It has been a life-long goal of mine. I've written things here and there over the years, but nothing ever came of them. I would start off super pumped, write a few chapters, and then I'd become too "busy" to finish the work I started. Other times, I'd just keep putting it off, saying that someday I'd finish.

But all of that changed when COVID-19 came into our lives and we found ourselves in the middle of a global pandemic. As I witnessed so much fear, loss, and uncertainty, I knew I could no longer keep assuming that I would have another tomorrow, especially since I work in the healthcare industry.

In my ten years of working in the caregiving industry, I've consistently received positive feedback. Most of my patients, and their family members, tell me the same thing: "I like *you* the best" or "*you*'re my favorite CNA." These comments always surprised me. Don't all CNAs get the same training? For the most part, yes. Don't all CNAs pass the same test? Pretty much yes. Don't all CNAs want to be caregivers? Mmm, not always. Don't all CNAs strive for the same thing? Well, not really. Don't we all have the tools to succeed? Yes, we do. Do we all use them appropriately? Probably not. There are so many reasons why some of us become CNAs, but there are some firm basic principles we need to follow to be successful ones.

This book is a combination of CNA best practices that I've learned over the years, real feedback that I've received from patients on what works for them, as well as feedback from colleagues, with time-saving tips that I wish that someone would have taught me when I first became an aide. The principles in this book are the daily practices that I live by and train other CNAs on, and if practiced consistently, each one will help set you apart and lift you up as an exemplary caregiver and human being. It is intended for anyone who is thinking about becoming a CNA, or individuals who are already CNAs and want to improve their job performance (think new career doors opening, better pay, job stability). But it's also for the directors of healthcare and caregiving facilities, who will learn about what tools we don't always have or know about, or how to achieve our goals sometimes we need their support, on the job training, and encouragement.

My hope for this book is to educate, inspire, and empower caregiving professionals to be the best that they can be in their work, as well as in their personal lives. With the proper knowledge, we can improve caregiving, one person and one company at a time.

— Christina Miles

PRINCIPLE 1

BE PUNCTUAL

The definition of punctuality is "the fact or quality of being on time." Being punctual is extremely important. I know that this might sound like an exaggeration, but it's true. *Why does it matter? Who cares if I show up to work five minutes late? It's only five minutes.*

For many, it doesn't seem like a big deal, but getting to work on time matters because it's a reflection of your character. Do you want to be known as the person who is always late? Or the person who is always on time? When you commit to working at a facility, or in an individual's home, you've entered into an agreement with your employer, your client, your colleagues, your patients, (and also yourself!), that you'll show up at the expected time of your shift.

You made a promise.

When you arrive to work on time, it shows others that they can depend on you, which results in people developing a greater level of trust and respect for you. When you're late, it not only affects *your* job performance but the performance of others as well. Let me show you how in the next few pages.

HOW PUNCTUALITY AFFECTS OTHERS

Lateness from Management's Perspective

When employees are late to work, it becomes the supervisor's problem. They have to stop what they're doing and figure out who hasn't arrived yet. Then, they need to see what wing or floor the missing employee is assigned to for that shift. And finally, they need to determine what patients were supposed to be cared for by that missing employee. The supervisor also needs to know if that CNA is actually coming to work or not. And if so, when will they arrive?

This interferes with your boss's already busy task load. Every moment spent dealing with staff who are tardy is critical time that could have been spent on more important matters, such as overseeing patient care.

Have you ever heard of the saying "Time is Money"? Well, that saying is also true. When employees are consistently late to work, it can cost a company thousands, sometimes even millions, of dollars a year due to their lack of productivity. "The flurry of activity caused by coming in late also throws others around them off focus, leading to a decrease in overall productivity in the office. Bottom line: As a business, you aren't getting what you pay for when an employee is consistently late and not doing their work-related tasks in a timely manner," states Lynda Moultry Belcher from the article "The Effect of Tardiness on Businesses." Now, some certified nursing assistants might not be bothered by this, and I can relate to why some may feel that way. The work that CNAs do is physically and emotionally challenging, and oftentimes we are overworked and underpaid. This can make anyone feel indifferent to the seriousness of the situation. But we have a choice, and we should always try to make the best out of the situation.

In the article "It's Staggering How Much Tardiness Cost the American Economy Each Year," on Inc.com, author Kenny Kline states "The reason employee tardiness can impact a company's economic standing is that chronic lateness frequently interferes with employee productivity." When an employee is consistently late to work, it decreases the facility's promise of quality care to its residents. This, in turn, causes paying residents, or their family members, to become dissatisfied or distrustful of the validity of the care they or their loved ones are receiving.

If patients or their family members are unhappy with the facility's services, they'll most likely do one of three things:

First, they'll leave and find another facility that's better equipped. This equals loss of income for a facility.

Second, they'll write negative reviews of their experience while at the facility. The chances of your name being mentioned in that review are high and might come up depending on the quality of care you provide to the patients. If your name does get mentioned in that negative review, it could result in you losing your job. But if you're doing a great job, your name will probably come up in the positive reviews.

Third, patients—or their family members—could sue a facility for neglect and lack of professional supervision that resulted in their loved one's pain, injury, substandard treatment, or recovery, just to name a few. All of these are not good scenarios and will hurt a facility's reputation, credibility, and financial standing.

So what does this have to do with me, Nina? I'm glad you asked. This can hurt *you* as well. If your employer is receiving negative reviews or is brought to court because of a lawsuit, this affects *everybody*. People will stop coming to be cared for at the company you work at, or they may be referred to a different facility instead. If you have fewer patients to care for, your hours will probably be reduced, or you may lose your job altogether. In the end, if your employer loses, you lose as well. How are you going to pay your mortgage, childcare, or college tuition then? Getting to work on time, and performing the tasks that are expected of you, when they are expected, is non-negotiable. It's what you signed up for.

Being late will also hinder your chances of career advancement. Your bosses will be less likely to choose you for a promotion or a raise if you have a poor attendance record. "As a leader, I'm always looking for talent. The employee who is consistently punctual stands out. They're demonstrating dependability. These are the people whom I'm going to give more opportunities and responsibilities to," says business leader Jon Rennie in his blog post "3 Reasons Why Punctuality Will Help Your Career." If you aren't offered better career opportunities due to your lateness, you may feel disappointed or frustrated. Watching your coworkers and friends advance while you stay in the same job position you started five years ago, making the same amount of money, isn't encouraging. It creates resentment.

If that's you, think for a moment about how much time you spent trying to find *that* job. Think about how much *you* invested, or are investing, into getting your certification, only to be put on the back burner when higher-paying career opportunities or promotions arise within the company, and you're never chosen because you're simply and consistently *late*.

For some people, working as a CNA might be just a temporary job until they find another career path. Or a stepping-stone to becoming a registered nurse. Either way, being punctual—no matter where you go in life—will always be important and will pay off in a positive way for you. Everyone will appreciate it.

Lateness from a Coworker's Perspective

When you regularly show up to work late, it creates an unstable and unfair work environment for your colleagues. At most facilities, you cannot leave until someone arrives to relieve you from your shift (change-of-shift report), so be mindful of that. The way I like to describe change-of-shift is like a relay race. Imagine there are two teams. The first team's runners are always there waiting, prepared at the starting line, ready to receive the baton from their teammate. That team is always consistent. The second team's runners sometimes are there to receive the baton from their teammates while other times they're late, they're distracted, or miss the handoff completely. That forces their teammates to then have to run a longer distance, faster, and do more work than they were originally supposed to. Which team do you think is going to be more productive and win more races? Also, which team members are going to have a better relationship with each other and be less stressed? Which team is going to feel more accomplished, happy, and supportive of each other? Think of that when it comes to getting to work on time. Do you arrive to work on time ready to receive the baton from your coworker, or are you the one who lets the baton fall and gets your teammates disqualified from the race?

Lastly, consider the single parent who had to drop her child off at her parent's house, stop to get gas on her way to work, and got caught in traffic, but who still managed to arrive at work on time. Only to find out when she gets to work that you're running late again because you overslept. Over time, this will cause discord and tension between you and your colleagues. Your coworker made it a priority to arrive at work on time and now they have to not only care for their own patients but yours as well until you finally show up to work. Simply put, it is not fair. Everyone is expected to be at work on time, and you're not exempt from this requirement.

Lateness from a Patient's or Family Member's Perspective

Change-of-shift is one of the busiest times in the caregiving industry. The previous staff members are leaving, and a new group of CNAs is beginning their shift. In my experience, change-of-shift is when the number of call bells ringing significantly increases. Residents will push their call bells for assistance, whether it's to receive medicine, go to the bathroom, or to see who the new caregiver is that will be taking care of them for the next eight-plus hours.

When employees are tardy, it leaves the on-site staff members (who came to work on time) and residents who need care, vulnerable to accidents. Your colleagues who arrived on time now have to care for twice the number of patients initially assigned to them, which creates stress. What's more, the residents must wait for longer periods of time to be cared for than usual because now your facility is short-staffed.

Patients will try to get up on their own and complete tasks for themselves if they feel that their call bell hasn't been answered in a timely manner or because they can no longer wait for assistance. Remember, if a resident has a fall prevention alarm, or has dementia, and tries on their own to walk, transfer themselves from bed to chair, or go to the bathroom on their own, this doubles the chances of an accident occurring. Many times, their actions result in them falling and getting injured, which is a very serious matter. That's why facilities go to great lengths to avoid this scenario from occurring. So again, please do your best to be at work on time for *everyone's* sake.

REAL-LIFE EXPERIENCE

One day I went into work for my regular scheduled shift, from 3:00 pm to 11:00 pm. At the last minute, someone called out (they couldn't come into work), and I was asked to stay and cover the overnight shift, from 11:00 pm to 7:00 am. I wasn't expecting to work a sixteen-hour shift, but I said yes so that my coworker would not have to work by himself, caring for twenty-plus residents on his own. So, I stayed.

What I thought would be an easy shift ended up being tougher than I had anticipated. The resident call bells rang nonstop all night long. As soon as I had gotten done answering and caring for one person, another resident was ringing for something else. The night seemed to never end. Finally, after a long day-and-a-half of work, 7:00 am rolled around, and I was thankful that soon I'd be able to go home and sleep! I began preparing my things, getting ready to leave. I stood at the nurse's station and waited with my belongings in one hand and the report sheet for the new aide coming in the other hand. My entire body was sore. Sweat was running down my back, my legs felt heavy as lead, and the soles of my feet were throbbing. I was drained! All I wanted to do was to go home, shower, eat, and crawl into bed, even if it meant that by the time I got to my room it would be 9:00 am. That would give me four hours of sleep. I had to be back at work at 3:00 pm later that day.

I watched anxiously as all the other day shift aides began to arrive. I waited patiently, but as time went on, my hope of freedom turned into anxiousness. My relief hadn't arrived. The shift change had come and passed, and I was the only aide from the night shift who was still at work. I tried to stay calm and think positively, but it was hard to do with all the resident call bells starting to ring nonstop again. My mind immediately went to all the negative "what ifs." *What if they were sick and weren't coming? What if they got into a car accident on the way to work and were now lying somewhere injured? And if that happened...what if they couldn't find someone to relieve me and I had to stay here another full shift?* I know I can be dramatic at times, but after sixteen hours of no sleep, your mind doesn't always think rationally.

When I had snapped out of it and came back to reality, I found a nurse calling the supervisor. He informed her that the unit was missing an aide and that I needed to be relieved ASAP. The supervisor had to stop what she was doing and had to start trying to find someone to pull from another floor so that I could leave. A few moments later, my relief strolled in at 7:15 am with a fast-food bag in one hand and an iced coffee from Dunkin' Donuts in the other. She was completely fine. Her explanation for being late was that the line at the drive-through was longer than she had expected.

PRACTICAL TIPS ON HOW TO BE PUNCTUAL

Calculate Your Drive Time.

You can download apps to your phone to help you find the fastest routes to work. Nowadays, you can calculate your drive time through apps like Google Maps, Waze, INRIX, MapQuest, etc. Find the fastest routes, especially if you're not familiar with the area you're going to, the neighborhood, or the facility. If it's the first time you're going to this job, ask what the parking situation is like for that specific location ahead of time, so you don't have to waste time trying to find a parking spot on top of everything else.

If you're running late to work, call your supervisor. Let them know when you'll arrive. It's proper etiquette and common courtesy.

Prepare Meals Before Work.

Being a CNA involves a lot of physical activity. Try to have healthy food options with you at all times so you can perform your job effectively. Make yourself a weekly meal plan. I highly suggest sitting down over the weekend and planning out all your meals for the upcoming week. You have no idea how much time this saves! Make a list of the items or ingredients you'll need to purchase at the grocery store, the cost, and the nutritional intake that each meal will provide your body. This will help you stay on budget and stay healthy at the same time.

Lay Out Work Clothes Ahead of Time.

To ensure that your clothes, uniform, or scrubs are always ready to wear for your next shift, lay them out the night before. Make sure your clothing is washed, stain-free, dry, *and* hanging in your room, ready for you, before you have to leave for work. There's nothing worse than having to leave in five minutes only to realize that you don't have any clean clothes to wear to work. Or that you forgot to put your scrubs in the dryer and they're sopping wet. This brings me to the next point.

Carry an Emergency Bag at All Times.

Pack a few tops, pants, underwear, socks, shoes, washcloths, a towel, toothbrush, toothpaste, and any shower supplies that you may need. This will come in handy if something unexpected ever happens at work and you need to change. Like the time a resident peed on me at work and I wasn't able to drive home (which was far away), to shower and change. My supervisor was only able to give me wet wipes and a hospital gown to complete my shift in. That was a long night and one that taught me a valuable lesson! Always be prepared for the unexpected.

Leave Your House Early.

Leave at least twenty minutes early and factor in unforeseeable events, such as:

Traffic

There's always going to be traffic somewhere, so leave early to avoid getting stuck in rush hour, behind school buses, or garbage trucks. Look up school bus schedules and garbage truck days and routes. It sounds like an exaggeration, I know, but doing this will save you a lot of time and stress. If you're taking the bus, keep a copy of the bus schedule handy, download your city's bus app on your phone, and sign up to get text alerts if your bus line is running late.

> **Carpool with a coworker whenever possible. It's a way to get to know someone and share the transportation cost.**

Construction

There's always a road being fixed somewhere. So do your best to figure out where the construction sites are and take a different route if possible. There's nothing worse than being very close to your work only to find yourself stuck in standstill construction traffic because a concrete truck is pouring cement fifty feet in front of you. If there's only one way to work—and I know there's construction in the area—I double my travel time and recalculate how long it will take me to get to my job. If I usually get to work in twenty minutes without construction, if there is construction, I'm going to need forty minutes. This always ensures that even when I get stuck in traffic, I'll still arrive to work early or on time.

Accidents

They're bound to happen and typically occur within a five-mile radius from your house or job. Become familiar with at least two or three other routes you can take. Learn about the area you're working in by looking at a map. You can Google your workplace on www.google. com/maps or ask colleagues who live in the area where you work for the best route advice. Ask them for information on backroads to take to get to and from work, learn about construction site prime times, or when the heavier traffic in that area occurs. For example, if a part of the city gets easily flooded when there is a storm, then you want to make sure to avoid those streets during the rainy season.

Holidays and Events

Remind yourself that national holidays, summer vacations, big sporting events, elections, concerts, protests, or rallies can all affect the traffic on your way to and from work. Calculate your driving route and leave your house early. It's better to get to work early and have to sit in your car than show up to work fifteen minutes late because there was an event you had forgotten about.

Bad Weather

Watch the news or check the weather app on your phone two hours before you have to leave for work. It could be sunny where you live but raining where your client's house or facility is located. Also, it's not a bad idea to become familiar with local hotels. If you get out of work after a long shift and are too tired or don't feel safe driving home in harsh weather, have a backup place where you can sleep in case of an emergency.

> If there's heavy rain, wind, or snow, leave your house an hour early.
>
> YOUR safety is the biggest priority.
>
> You won't be able to care for anyone if you're injured or hurt.

HELPFUL RESOURCES

"How to Be On Time Every Time"
article by Dustin Wax on Lifehack.org

"The Importance of Being on Time for Work"
article by Ruth Mayhew on Careertrend.com

"3 Reasons Why Punctuality Will Help your Career (Time Management)"
article by Jon Rennie on leadx.org

Time Management: Perfecting the Lifestyle Called Punctuality: Become Time-Conscious Before It's Too Late
book by Jeremy Bolton

"The Importance of Being Punctual"
YouTube video by Richard Crenian

PERSONAL COMMITMENT

These are the three things I commit to working on
to improve my punctuality:

1. _____

2. _____

3. _____

Date: _____ My Signature: _____

PRINCIPLE 2

PRIORITIZE YOUR HEALTH

Having good health is crucial when it comes to being a certified nursing assistant. Oxford Dictionary defines health as "the state of being free from illness or injury." You have to take care of yourself first to be able to take care of others. It's like what they tell parents on airplanes: Put the oxygen mask on yourself *first* and *then* put it on your child. Not the other way around. If you're not in good health, how are you going to help others who rely on you to care for them? You won't be able to.

Prioritizing your health, physically, mentally, and financially is vital because being a CNA is a strenuous profession. It's physically and emotionally demanding. It requires "all of you" to be there. CNAs are the group most at risk of getting injured within the healthcare industry. According to a 2012 article by Laura Walter on EHS Today[1], "60 percent of certified nursing assistants (CNAs) employed in nursing homes incur occupational injuries."

---

1. https://www.ehstoday.com/health/article/21915146/60-percent-of-nursing-assistants-in-nursing-homes-incur-occupational-injuries

More than half of all aides will get injured at some point in time during their careers. This is a startling statistic but believe it or not, it's true. The most common injuries aides get while on the job are back and shoulder injuries; often they'll experience joint pain, and aides may even develop arthritis. I know this statistic to be true because it also happened to me. I was transferring a patient, and in a single movement, my mobility, health, independence, and financial security were jeopardized. A shooting pain ran from the top of my lower back all the way down the back of my leg. The pain was so intense that it knocked the wind out of me, and I almost fell over. Within the next couple of weeks, I had to take off work, see several doctors, took medication around the clock, and had to do physical therapy at home until I recovered. It was not fun for myself nor for my mom who had to help take care of me during that time that I was laid up.

Managing your emotional health, along with your nutritional intake, is just as important as your physical well-being. Maybe even more so. There's a lot of stress that goes along with the job, and responsibly managing what you eat will also help you succeed in your career. You want to be in the best health possible so that you can be there for your patients, their family members, your colleagues, your supervisors, as well as your family. They're all counting on you.

HOW YOUR HEALTH AFFECTS OTHERS

Your Health from Management's Perspective

When an employee gets injured on the job, it not only puts a physical strain on a company (because it's now missing an able-bodied person to provide hands-on care to their patients) but a financial one as well.

Every time a certified nursing assistant gets hurt at work a facility has to provide their employee with Workers' Compensation by law. This can be costly, and it's a long, bureaucratic process to go through. Many times, aides that are injured may be required to do "light duty" which is a fancy way of saying "menial tasks." But every facility is different. "Light responsibilities" can range from desk work, charting, dusting, to cleaning a facility.

When I had my back injury, I was put on "light duty," which required me to work in the basement for eight hours a day, folding towels and washcloths. That ended up hurting my back even more because of the long hours and fast-paced, repetitive motions required sometimes in housekeeping. Eventually, because my condition was getting worse, my doctor provided me with a note requesting that I be allowed to recover at home instead of in the company's laundry room. Even though I was out of work for a few weeks, I was grateful to at least qualify for Worker's Compensation and get a percentage of my wages. But remember, worker's comp is not free money. There are no big payouts and cheaters are eventually caught (insurance companies can make home visits and do surveillance if they suspect someone is lying). Workers' Compensation fraud can even lead to time in jail.

If you consider the quote I mentioned earlier and think that one facility may have 60% of their aides, at some point in time, getting injured, that's a lot of money to pay for every CNA who gets hurt while at work. Your employer does their best to ensure that their staff stays safe and healthy, but someone will inevitably get hurt. And that someone, more often than not, is usually going to be a CNA. Strive to be part of the 40% of CNAs who do not get injured at work. Do this by prioritizing your health.

LeBron James's former teammate, Mike Miller, said James treats his body like an *investment*. LeBron James reportedly spends 1.5 million dollars a year to take care of his body. That includes his home gym, trainers, massage therapists, chefs, appliances, and more. You definitely don't need to spend that much but imagine how unstoppable you could be if you just focused on improving one area of your health at a time such as eating, sleeping, exercising, increasing your water intake, becoming financially independent, or even getting counseling. Just commit to it for ninety days and see how you feel at the end. It will not only help *you* but also help those *around* you.

Your Health from a Coworker's Perspective

Your health not only affects you but your colleagues as well. If you're not feeling well often or are constantly calling-out sick, you're putting your coworkers at a disadvantage. Now I know that getting sick or injured is out of anyone's control for the most part, but there are many things you can do to reduce the risk of this occurring.

I once worked with an aide who would stay up late every night binge-watching his favorite TV shows. Whenever I would work with him, he was always exhausted. He would yawn constantly, and it always took him a long time to answer his patients' call bells because he was mentally and physically exhausted. That's not a clever way to work your shift. Lack of sleep is something that he could have controlled. Staying up late was his choice, but it was a poor decision, and it affected all of us that worked with him. When you're not on your A game, it forces your colleagues to carry a heavier load than they already have to. It's unfair and it can for the most part be avoided.

In contrast to that, I have a colleague whom I love to work with because she always comes to work on her A game. She's well-rested and this enables her to be full of energy, spread good vibes, and care for her patients in a timely manner. This makes the shift go by a lot smoother. I know I can rely on her and it's a huge relief because I know I'll be able to get my own work done too. You want to be the kind of colleague that others can rely on to do their job. There is nothing more infuriating than having to keep cleaning up someone else's mess because they don't have their act together. To make poor decisions once in a blue moon is okay, we are all human, but weekly occurrences are unacceptable. Especially if you keep making the same wrong decisions over and over again. We must all do our fair share of work, and you can't do that if you're continually feeling ill or are tired all the time. Focusing on your health should be your number one priority.

Your Health from a Patient's or Family Member's Perspective

Believe it or not, residents can tell when you're not feeling well or when you aren't on your A game. I don't know how, but they can always sense it. And what happens next? It can cause anxiousness or fear in a patient and their family members. I can't tell you the number of times I wasn't feeling well, and a patient would ask me if I was okay because I looked tired or sick. Think about it, no one wants a sick, injured, or tired person to take care of them. You might be putting their life or health at risk. You must take proper care of yourself daily. Being a certified nursing assistant is not just a job but it's a service one provides to *others*. To perform that service efficiently and effectively you have to be mindful of your health. You must take it seriously and prioritize it above the other things going on in your life.

REAL-LIFE EXPERIENCE

One day I was in a patient's room helping the nurse with a dressing change when all of a sudden, boom! I collapsed onto the floor. A few minutes later, when I regained consciousness, I awoke to chaos. I had fainted, the nurse was distressed, and the patient was freaking out. They were calling my name, asking me if I was alright, and had pushed the patient's call button to get someone in the room to assist me. It took a few moments of me sitting upright against the wall before I felt stable enough to stand up. Although the nurse and patient were very worried, I was okay, just embarrassed because I had brought this on myself. The reason I fainted was my own fault. I hadn't eaten or drunk anything all day. I'd woken up late, rushed out the door without having breakfast or lunch, and then worked an eight-hour shift on an empty stomach. Not smart. It never looks good when the person who is caring for you is the one who gets sick. I learned my lesson. Always prioritize your health please!

After that experience, I began focusing on correcting my poor eating habits and diet. I started planning my meals before work. I learned that our health is made up of 80% of what we eat and 20% of getting the right type of exercise for our body and age.

PRACTICAL TIPS ON HOW TO PRIORITIZE YOUR HEALTH

Choose Foods that Nourish Your Body

I love the saying, "What you eat is what you'll become." When it comes to eating healthy, don't think of it in terms of weight. That's not what I'm talking about. It's not about dieting or trying to lose weight. You should be thinking of it in terms of making the inside of your body as strong and healthy as possible. How do you do that? By eating a balanced diet made up of a variety of foods that will strengthen your immune system while also giving you energy. The key word being *variety*.

Your body is a high functioning machine that should only be consuming the best fuel. Trust me, I know that this can be difficult. I've been struggling with the ramifications of my unhealthy eating habits since adolescence. It may not look like it because I'm petite but being skinny doesn't mean being healthy. For some people, poor diet habits show in their waist size, but for me, my unhealthy food choices show up as painful acne bumps and dark spots all over my face.

Change is difficult, especially when it's for the better. If you know that you need to change your eating habits, but don't know where to start, ask your doctor or a certified nutritionist. As we age and our bodies change, our bodies need different nutritional intakes, different vitamins or supplements, different exercises. What worked in our twenties may not work in our forties or in our sixties. Once you have the right information, make a meal and exercise plan. Find an accountability partner that can help you stay on course. Try to make this experience fun and simple. Share new recipes you discover with your friends, colleagues, partners, and children. **Remember, this is a long and slow journey you're embarking on, not a sprint, so be graceful and patient with yourself.** It will be worth it in the long run.

Drink Lots of Water

One of my all-time favorite motivational speakers is Rachel Hollis, who suggests drinking half of your body weight in ounces of water, daily. For example, I weigh about one-hundred pounds, so my goal each day is to drink about fifty ounces of water per day (approximately three seventeen-ounce bottles, or six large cups). Disclaimer: when you drink that much water a day, you're going to pee a lot. But that's a good thing! Just make sure you know where the nearest bathroom is at all times. It may be annoying at the beginning, but every time you pee, you're ridding your body of toxins and things your body no longer needs (and thank your kidneys for that!)

Take Your Vitamins and Supplements

This is crucial to living a long and healthy life. Throughout our lives, many of us will be deficient in one vitamin or another. That's why eating a variety of foods ("eating the rainbow") is so important to get all the vitamins we need. But sometimes our bodies don't create enough of one vitamin or don't create it at all. The best way to learn about what your body needs is to ask your doctor. They'll make sure to recommend the correct ones that are going to help you feel and live your best life. Ask if you should take liquid vitamins (which some medical professionals say are better absorbed by the body) or tablet ones. Ask what the right time of day to take them is (many recommend taking them at night, when your body is resting, for better absorption). Remember, we are all different and don't need to take the same kinds of vitamins. What is best for me, might not be what is best for you. Again, this is YOUR HEALTH JOURNEY.

Sleep

Sleep and rest—two different things—are essential for your body to create energy. If you have energy, you feel refreshed and alert, you strengthen your immune system, which in turn helps your body fight off illnesses. If you aren't getting enough sleep, you're putting yourself at a disadvantage. The Sleep Foundation compares not getting enough sleep to feeling jet lagged. Who wants to go through their day feeling like that? Not me. I've struggled with sleep deprivation for many years and it truly feels miserable. Not getting enough sleep can lead to feelings of depression, anger, anxiousness, and frustration. Feelings you don't need to encourage if you're already working in a stressful environment.

The goal of staying healthy is to decrease your stress levels, not increase them. Set a regular bedtime for yourself (yes, like a child!) Try not to eat right before you go to bed so your body is not triggering your digestive system to work instead of rest. Try not to watch TV right before going to bed. And don't sleep with your phone! I know. I can feel your glares coming my way. I'm here to help and encourage you to make positive health choices that are within your reach! Reducing all these things will help you to have a better night's sleep, and the feeling of waking up rested is priceless. If you work nights, get an eye mask and dark curtains for your room to block out the sunlight. Turn your phone completely off or activate its "do not disturb feature" for the hours you plan to sleep.

Exercise

You can do this alone or with a buddy to do it with. Make it fun! Exercising with another person can make it easier *and more* enjoyable. Also, exercise at the same time every day, that way your body gets into a routine. Many people feel it's easier to tack exercise onto an existing habit. Start with twenty minutes. Then slowly increment that. PBS's Miranda Esmonde-White has some great free easy workouts on YouTube that will get you moving and feeling better in no time.

Walk

Go on a walk for fifteen minutes a day. And no, the treadmill doesn't count! You want to be outside in nature or cruising through the green parts of your city. Breathing in fresh air and experiencing all of nature's elements through your five senses is energizing. This is a great time if you're an introvert like me to listen to a podcast and have some alone time. Or if you're an extrovert, use this time to catch up with a friend as you both walk around the block. During COVID-19 times, my friend Linda goes on socially distant walks with a neighbor three nights a week. They call each other on the phone to talk, but walk together, on opposite sidewalks, for forty-five minutes. Linda says that after each walk, she feels physically and mentally rejuvenated and that time flies when engaged in deep conversation.

Stretch

Stretching is extremely important. The goal of stretching is to loosen your muscles gently. Let me emphasize the word *gently*! Stretching also keeps your muscles flexible, strong, and healthy. Miranda Esmonde-

White has some great beginner workouts to help stretch and hydrate your connective tissue as well. We usually forget about our connective tissue, but it's what holds the structure of our body together. We need to be stretching this part of our body as well!

Meditate

This can mean different things to different people. Some people will instantly think of yoga's "Lotus pose" (*Padmasana*) and gentle breathing exercises. However, for others, it means chanting or sitting in nature. But when I think about meditating, I think of "journaling." Putting all my thoughts, fears, concerns, and joys down on paper. This helps me clear my mind. Find what works for you and commit to doing it for fifteen minutes a day.

Have Fun

Find a hobby that's outside of work. Socialize! Connect with other human beings and talk about other things that aren't work-related. If you're an introvert, socializing may not be your thing, but reach out to someone with whom you enjoy talking to or doing things with. Also, plan trips or scenic drives. It doesn't have to be far or expensive but think of fun day trips you can do on your day off once a month. Shake things up, have fun, and explore new places and activities. Even during these difficult pandemic times, there are things you can do safely without putting your health, or someone else's, at risk. You only live once, and you don't want to look back when you're retired and realize that all you did your entire life was work. Strive to have a good work-life balance. You'll be happier now, and you'll be happier later too.

Talk to Someone

Working in the caregiving profession can be emotionally draining, even if sometimes we are not aware of the effect it is having on our own lives. We are constantly seeing people who are hurt, who suffer from memory loss or physical ailments, as well as patients without family members nearby who can provide them with love and emotional support. And on a daily basis, we even see death.

All this can have a very heavy emotional toll on you as a caregiver. You should never try to bear all this weight alone. And all of us have personal lives, with families or friends that we also care for, so we also need to stay "mind-healthy." Don't be discouraged if you're feeling anxiety, depression, stress, or agitation. Those are normal *and* human feelings. And there are many (free) ways to cope with them. The World Health Organization (WHO) released a document in March of 2020 with advice on protecting your mental health during the coronavirus outbreak. Much of what they advocate for applies just as well during "normal" times.

The BBC has summarized the information into five steps:

1. Limit the news and be careful of what you read

2. Take breaks from social media and mute things/people that are triggering

3. Stay connected with people, especially those you care about. Ask a friend to check in with you weekly. Or reach out to them. "Hey, I could really use five minutes to talk" is a phrase most friends or family members welcome

4. Keep a routine, or start a new one

5. Avoid burnout or anxiety with the "Apple" technique:

"A"   Acknowledge any uncertainty or issues that are coming up for you

"P"   Pause and breathe, don't react as you normally do

"P"   Pull back, remember it's only a thought or a feeling. Thoughts are not statements or facts.

"L"   Let go of the thought or feeling. Remind yourself "this will pass." You don't always need to respond to a feeling. Imagine it floating away.

"E"   Explore the present moment. What do you see, feel, hear, smell? Shift your focus to something else.

And if all of that isn't enough, please reach out and get help. There is a community of professionals who have studied and work with these feelings every-single-day. You matter. Your work matters. We need more people like you in the world, so please take care of yourself. We all care about you.

Your Financial Health

For the last few years, I've been working on improving my financial health, but it wasn't until the last year that my mindset around the matter shifted. I no longer had the luxury of financial procrastination. For months I had been telling myself that I would devote my time to learning how to make my money work for me and not the other way around, but that never happened. I would always put it off until tomorrow. A lot of tomorrows came and went, and I still hadn't become any financially better off than I was before I became a CNA. It wasn't until I saw how COVID-19 stole so many people's lives, health, and financial security that I realized I could no longer wait to become financially healthy.

I would challenge every person reading this book to do the same. In the caregiving industry, CNAs get paid very low wages so it's crucial to be in control of your finances at all times. Newsflash: No one else is going to do this for you. No one else is going to set money aside for you. No one else is going to figure out how to make *you* successful. You have to do it and commit to it yourself. Try not to live paycheck to paycheck. Most of us start off that way, but it creates unnecessary stress that you don't need. Knowing you have planned for your financial future and that you're setting—even a tiny bit—of money aside (for emergencies, a trip you want to take, a more reliable car you want to buy, a conference you want to go to, a new laptop you might need, or funds for retirement) will help you sleep better at night.

It's easy to start, trust me! You can do this in parts during your lunch break. First, grab a notebook and write down all the things you spend money on, and how much, in a given month:

- Housing (rent, mortgage)
- Transportation (car payment, auto insurance, gas, bus pass)
- Food (groceries, take out, vending machines—you *can* control your food expenses)
- Childcare
- Cell phone
- Health Insurance

- Debt payments (always pay on time and try to get rid of these asap. If you've been paying on time, call your credit card company to get a lower APR)
- Utilities (electricity, gas, water, trash)
- Entertainment (apps, TV subscriptions, hobbies, sporting events—this is where most overspending occurs)
- Clothing
- Grooming (hair, nails, cosmetics)

Keep track of these expenses every month and tally up how much you're spending overall. Ask yourself, are you happy with how you are managing your money? Or can you do better? The good news is that YOU DO have the ability and power to improve your financial health. Of all the expenses above, it's really easy to trim food, grooming, and for sure entertainment. See how much you're spending on those things now and set a goal of reducing each one of them a bit every week.

Then, if you already have a checking account, get a savings account (they're usually free) and transfer that amount you're saving each week on those expenses to your savings account. After a few weeks of this, you'll be surprised at how much you're able to set aside for yourself. Be strong and keep that money in there, don't touch it unless absolutely necessary. If you don't have a checking account, then grab that cash you're saving and put it in a piggy bank for adults (yes, they do exist!) Promise yourself not to open it until six months have passed. If you get to the six months mark, try keeping it there for another six months, and so on.

Learn to invest your money so it can accumulate over time and multiply. I've lived paycheck to paycheck for several years until

I decided no more. I want to create wealth for not only myself but my parents and future children as well. If you're like me and have the "entrepreneur bug" and want to create financial wealth, generate passive income, and become financially healthy but don't know where to start, here are some videos that I've found helpful:

Patricia Bright's YouTube The Break Channel talks about how to manage your salary and budget better. Her energy and drive are inspiring! Suze Orman's book *The Money Book for the Young, Fabulous & Broke* talks about how us younger generations need to learn to handle our finances better with solutions to common problems. I also respect the work of Dave Ramsey in his book *The Total Money Makeover: A Proven Plan for Financial Fitness* and *Smart Women Finish Rich* by David Bach. Lastly, Anthony ONeal's *Destroy Your Student Loan Debt* is a great resource for those of us managing our student debt.

Remember, most of these books you can get for free from your local library, or in audiobook format so you can listen to them while driving, folding laundry, or doing the dishes. It is never too late to start working on improving your financial health so that you can live the life that you deserve.

Be Thankful

Gratitude is such a beneficial practice. It's so easy to focus on all the things in our life that are going wrong, that we seldom take a step back to reflect on the good things that we have or that have happened to us. Whether it's through meditation, prayer, or simply taking five minutes out of your day to acknowledge the positives in your life, it's an excellent practice.

HELPFUL RESOURCES

"10 Best Ways to Stay Healthy as a CNA"
article by cnalicense.org

"How to budget money: Tackle your debt and start saving"
article by Matthew Goldberg

"30-Minute Hip-Hop Tabata to Torch Calories"
YouTube video by "POPSUGAR Fitness"

"20 min workout at home for beginners | full body/ no equipment"
YouTube video, Daniela Suarez

"The Relationship Between Sleep and Industrial Accidents"
article by SleepFoundation.org

"Gratitude Journal: A Collection of 67 Templates,
Ideas and Apps for Your Diary"
journal ideas on how to start and keep a gratitude journal
by Courtney E. Ackerman, MSc. of PositivePsychology.com

PERSONAL COMMITMENT

These are the three things I commit to doing
to improve my overall health:

1. _____

2. _____

3. _____

Date: _____ My Signature: _____

PRINCIPLE 3

FINE TUNE YOUR COMMUNICATION SKILLS

Having good communication skills is vital for a certified nursing assistant. Being able to communicate with others effectively (saying what you mean) and efficiently (without wasting time) will help you succeed in your professional career and also throughout your life.

Communication is simply the act of transferring information from one person, place, or group to another. A **sender** and a **recipient.** *Why does it matter? What does any of this have to do with providing care to someone?* That's a great question! Thank you for asking. Having exceptional communication skills may sound simple, even easy, but it's actually very complex. Just because we know how to talk doesn't mean we know how to *communicate.*

Try to improve your communication skills with others on a daily basis. Being a good communicator is active work. Do you know that you spend 50%–80% of your day communicating with others, and others with you, directly or indirectly? Whether it's sending a text message, responding to an email, listening to a podcast, giving a speech, watching a presentation online, or using nonverbal gestures (such as your body language), all of these are forms of communication.

Having good communication skills is by far, one of the most valuable gifts we possess as human beings. If you're not communicating correctly, what you have to say may not be understood. Or worse yet, it might be misunderstood, which is never a good thing, especially when working in the caregiving industry. We've all been there when we think we said something clearly, but the message came across completely wrong. *Yeah, I know all of this, but what does this have to do with me and my job, Nina?* Let me show you.

HOW COMMUNICATION AFFECTS OTHERS

Communication from Management's Perspective

In the article "Measurement of Time Spent Communicating," research done by the McKinsey Global Institute, International Data Corporation, and the Journal of Communication, found that "Leaders spend 50%-80% of the workday communicating." Management spends 28% of their day reading and responding to emails, 26% of the day on the phone. Senior management spends 50% of their workday time in meetings. That's a lot of communicating! With your bosses being so busy dealing with patients and their family members, resident care, staffing issues, annual budgets, billing, insurance claims, etc., the last thing they want to deal with is another problem. Especially if it's a problem coming from low on the totem pole. That's where you and

I come in my friend. In the medical world, certified nursing assistants are the lowest step on the ladder. If you can eliminate yourself from being a problem, that will take a lot of stress off your employer, which in turn will help *you* in the long run.

I'm sure that there's someone in your close circle that's always responsible and mindful, that you never have to worry about. Whether it's your child, a parent, a friend, student, or significant other, you know that there could be a hundred problems happening in a day, but they will not be one of them. Your colleagues and supervisors at work should feel the same about you. You should be communicating with them on a daily basis, and they should know they can rely on you because you'll be doing your job as expected.

Side Note: Let's make this very clear, **your boss is NOT your friend.** Don't get this twisted. You shouldn't be texting them unless it's absolutely necessary. And you should ask for permission to text them. NEVER text them about your personal matters, unless it's something that's going to interfere with you performing your job. Always keep things professional.

Here are some things you *should* be communicating to management or your supervisor about in a timely manner:

- If you're running late or have to leave early

- If you have to call out try to give six or more hours of notice *before* your scheduled shift. Don't wait until the last minute. (See your company's guidelines for their policy on this)

- If you, or a family member, is sick enough to warrant having to go to the doctor. (A hangover, headache, or cramps doesn't count unless you're injured.) Remember that's a sick day you could have used wisely instead

- Family emergencies: When a death or a family crisis occurs, that hinders your availability to work

- If you have a serious medical history or condition(s) that could get worse at work and be a health risk for you, your patients, your coworkers, or your employer (pregnancy, asthma, heart conditions, chronic back pain, migraines, fainting spells, diabetes, or seizures)[2]

- Future vacations or dates that you'll be unavailable to work. Try to give your supervisor, boss, or HR, two or more months of advanced, written notice of the dates you need off

- Religious holidays or practices. Again, give as much advanced notice as possible

Read your company's policy for how to properly address "sick leave," "personal leave," "paid time off," and "vacation days" because you may have to provide written documentation to your employer. It's always good to do so if you can. Why written? Because you want to have that documented proof that you informed someone in management for your own protection. Having a conversation doesn't count. Unless you have it in writing on a piece of paper, or in an email, that has your name on it, the conversation never took place. This is very important! Trust me, I learned this lesson the hard way and I want to spare you of what I had to go through. It also makes you look professional and it tells your supervisors that you value your job and take it seriously.

---

2. If you take medications for any of these conditions always carry them with you to minimize exacerbations at work and inform your employer of your medical condition.

Please communicate your absences to your boss or employer. It's common courtesy and they'll appreciate you for it.

Research has shown that there "is a clear connection between effective communication and a company's bottom line" states Noah Zandan, CEO of Quantifiedcommunications.com, a communication performance platform. In a company of just a hundred employees, an employer spends an average of seventeen hours a week correcting or clarifying miscommunication that occurred the previous week. *That's interesting Nina, but why does that matter? How does it affect us CNAs?* Your miscommunications could cost your employer hundreds of thousands of dollars a year, plus significantly aggravating your boss and coworkers, which could result in you being fired from your job because of your mistakes and inability to *clearly* communicate.

You don't want to be that person.

Don't be part of the problem, be part of the solution.

Make sure that you're communicating concise and factual information to your employer, so they don't have to waste time double-checking it. Also, if you're not sure about something, that's okay. Just ask! We are not expected to be walking encyclopedias or technical manuals. Asking questions and listening to the responses you're given is just as essential as verbal and written communication. Make sure everything is clear to you. Never assume! A great technique you can use is that after you've been told something new and you're not sure that you understood the information correctly, repeat it back to the person who explained it to you. This is called "active listening." And if you become a pro at it, everyone will appreciate the effort you're making.

Communication from a Coworker's Perspective

Creating a strong foundation of communication with your colleagues is crucial. I don't know how to stress this enough. Your coworkers are the ones who have your back at work, so you need to be on good terms with them. Now, this doesn't mean that you have to be best friends or even *friends* with the people that you work with, but it does mean that you should be cordial with your colleagues. Keep things professional. There isn't time for petty nonsense. You're there to provide care to your patients. They're relying on you. This should be the only thing that matters. If you have a problem with someone that you work with, particularly another aide, try to resolve the matter as soon as possible. First, try to handle it yourself with the other individual. If the problem continues, gets worse, or if it's putting a resident's safety at risk, then go to your supervisor. This should be a last resort. Again, you don't want to be one of your boss's problems.

Here are things that you should be communicating to your coworkers on every shift:

- If you have to care for a patient for an extended time

- If you're stepping off of the floor, wing, or unit, and for how long

- If you need help with a patient

- When you're going on break and what time you'll be back

- What assignment, cart, or wing you'll be working on

- If you're feeling unwell or have to leave your shift early due to an unforeseen emergency

- The status of your residents

- Which residents are incontinent, which are at risk of falling, which patients require two or more people to be transferred

- Which patient isn't feeling well, who has serious medical conditions

- Which residents are on fluid restrictions, or on special diets

Get into the habit of communicating as much as possible.

Communication is key to creating a pleasant and reliable work environment.

Communication from a Patient's or Family Member's Perspective

I've found that the core reason why a lot of patients or their family members get upset is that there is a lack of communication with them from employees, and between employees. I strongly believe it's better to "over communicate" than to "under communicate." A patient once told me that they wanted to be *talked to* and not *talked at*. I think that's something that we all share in common. If you explain things to your patients and their families beforehand, more often than not they'll be understanding and work with you instead of fighting with you about it. In the end, you and the patient both want the same thing. The residents want to be properly cared for, and you want your patients to stay healthy, safe, and accident-free. All of which is possible through effective communication!

REAL-LIFE EXPERIENCE

One evening I went into work and before starting my shift I asked the CNA who worked the previous shift how everything went that day. She gave me the generic "Everyone is good!" response and left.

I took her at her word and began doing my rounds, checking on all the patients who were assigned to me. Everything was going smoothly until halfway through my shift. One of my residents asked me for a snack, so I gave them a handful of treats and beverages. Fifteen minutes later, when I went back in to check on the patient, they were having a difficult time breathing. I immediately got the nurse. When the nurse entered, they were horrified to see all the empty wrappers and the soda can lying on the resident's tray table. The nurse sprang into action. She checked the resident's vital signs. They were abnormal. The nurse instructed me to go and get her coworker who was working on another medicine cart down the hall. I ran out of the room and got the nurse. After a few minutes, they were able to stabilize the patient, but it was a close call.

I was later brought into the supervisor's office and scolded for giving "regular food" to a patient who was on a special diet and thickened liquids (their diet had been downgraded).

"Didn't M tell you that the doctor downgraded Mrs. P's diet today when she gave you the report?" asked the director of nursing.

"No, I had no idea! Otherwise, I wouldn't have given Mrs. P the snacks!" I replied.

"Well, I told her to tell you that Mrs. P, was placed on new diet restrictions," said the director of nursing in frustration.

Thankfully, the resident was okay, but it could have ended very badly for everyone involved. The nurse and I had to write lengthy personal statements as to what occurred, and it was brought to management's attention. We both got in trouble for the incident. The next day when the aide was asked by the director of nursing why they hadn't passed the information along to me about Mrs. P's diet being downgraded, her response was, "Oh shit, I forgot!"

Good communication is not only fundamental, but it SAVES LIVES.

PRACTICAL TIPS ON HOW TO IMPROVE YOUR COMMUNICATION

Practice Talking to Yourself in a Mirror.

I know that this may seem silly but talking to yourself in a mirror will help to see yourself speaking. Being able to observe what your facial expressions are while you speak is very helpful. I used this technique a lot when I first became a CNA because a lot of the residents kept commenting that I looked afraid or unsure of myself while I was talking to them, so I began practicing in the mirror every day. The more I practiced the more confident I became. The residents were thankful for the improvement.

Speak to Yourself Out Loud.

Again, I know this may seem unnatural or uncomfortable, but it will help you to become comfortable with hearing the sound of your own voice—the way that you enunciate certain words, how to improve inflections, and how the tone of your voice sounds. I've had to practice long and hard when it came to this one as well. When I was a child, I was painfully shy, and I didn't speak unless spoken to. Because of that, it became hard for me to speak to anyone who wasn't a family member. So, when I got older, I knew that if I was ever going to succeed in life, I had to improve my communication skills. When I'd overcome my fear of speaking to strangers, I then began working on increasing the volume level of my voice. This was also very challenging for me, but it was necessary if I wanted to do my job well. I've always been very soft-spoken, but that doesn't work when you're caring for residents who are hard of hearing. I had to become comfortable with being uncomfortable. I can still remember the first day that I felt brave enough to practice at work. I felt as though I was yelling at my patients, but in reality, I wasn't. My throat hurt like hell the next day from all the practicing. I just wasn't used to raising my voice to that level before and for so many hours. But my patients noticed, and they appreciated my improvement. **I had to adjust my communication style so that I could effectively communicate with my patients and colleagues, even if it made me uncomfortable.**

Know When to Ask Questions and When to Listen.

Don't be afraid. If you're unsure of something, please ask. Especially when it comes to working in caregiving. That's the simplest way to reduce misinformation or mistakes from occurring. Your supervisor will appreciate that you're trying to accurately understand the situation or instructions you've been given. I know that this may seem easy, or obvious, but many times it can be quite difficult.

Other times people just want to be heard without having you say anything back to them. One time a patient confided in me about a difficult personal matter they were going through, and I didn't say a word. I just sat there and held their hand while they talked for ten minutes. That's all they needed from me. They wanted someone to be present and listen to them, and what they needed from me was my company and my silence.

Body Language.

This is just as pertinent to understand as verbal communication is. Your body language behavior is made up of your facial expressions, the gestures you make, your eye movement, your posture, your touch, and how you use the space around you. You'll need to learn how to talk to patients that have intellectual delay, residents who don't speak English, patients whose hearing and speech are impaired, or people who have any other physical impediment that would interfere with communication. The Royal College of Nursing has a section of their website dedicated to nonverbal communication that's very insightful (see the resources section below).

Check Your Writing!

Always proofread anything you've written before handing it in. When I write something down that has to be reviewed by a nurse or management, I make sure to triple-check what I've written. Then I have someone else check it as well before handing it in. It's a good habit to get into. If you're filling out a form, a good exercise is to check it backward. Start at the end of the form and make your way to the beginning to make sure you haven't missed anything. If you're reporting an incident, remember to answer to the best of your ability the "5 Ws and 1 H," which means, make sure you're stating Who, What, When, Where, Why and How something happened. By doing this, I reduce the possibility of errors and misinformation that I'm turning in, and it makes me look more professional. It also shows that I care about my work and take it seriously. Remember, everyone makes mistakes, but if you ask for help, you have the opportunity to correct and learn from them.

HELPFUL RESOURCES

"4 Types Of Communication (With Examples)"
YouTube video by Jen, Career Coach at Indeed.com

Royal College of Nursing, nonverbal communication, website

"Communication skills 3: non-verbal communication"
article by Nursing Times

"Effective Communication in the Workplace: How and Why?"
article by Vartika Kashyap

"13 Reasons Why Workplace Communication Matters"
article by Nozomi Morgan

"The Importance of Effective Communication in the Workplace"
article by Joanna Zambas

4 Essential Keys to Effectively Communicate in Love, Life, Work--Anywhere!
book by Bento C. Leal III

PERSONAL COMMITMENT

These are the three things I commit to doing
to improve my communication skills:

1. _____

2. _____

3. _____

Date: _____ My Signature: _____

PRINCIPLE 4

BE A TEAM PLAYER

Phil Jackson, the great American professional basketball player, head coach, and executive director, once said, "Good teams become great ones when the members trust each other enough to surrender the Me for the We." I cannot stress the importance of teamwork enough. The definition of teamwork by Merriam-Webster Dictionary is "work done by several associates with each doing a part but all subordinating personal prominence to the efficiency of the whole." What that definition is saying is that everyone knows what their specific role is. Still, every person comes together to fulfill the company's overall goal and/or mission. In the healthcare industry, the overall mission is for caregiving workers to provide their patients with exceptional quality care.

"Alone we can do so little, together we can do so much."

HELEN KELLER

Being a team player is crucial when working as a CNA. If you don't collaborate with your colleagues, patients, and bosses, it will make your job even more stressful and challenging than it already is.

"Together, ordinary people can achieve extraordinary results."
BECKA SCHOETTLE.

Some of you are probably thinking to yourself, *"Cool. Play nice with your coworkers. I get it!"* That's great. I'm so happy to hear that! Sounds easy, right? That's until you realize that everyone at work is different. We come from different cultural backgrounds, we have different values and beliefs, we grew up differently, we like different things. So just in case anyone doesn't understand how to make the team effort work, and why it's of the essence, here are some thoughts to get your ideas going.

HOW BEING A TEAM PLAYER AFFECTS OTHERS

Being a Team Player from Management's Perspective

In the healthcare industry, most facilities have a person, or a department, whose sole purpose is to prepare the shift schedules for all personnel. Scheduling is done so that resources (doctors, nurses, CNAs, rooms, equipment, medicines) match the patient's needs. Though usually hidden in a back office, their job is crucial to helping an organization run smoothly, allocating staff when and where they're needed *ahead of time.*

When the scheduler of a facility, hospital, nursing, or retirement home is staffing a unit, they look at the ratio of patients that need to be cared for and the number of employees they'll need to care for those patients. *Sure, OK, but what does any of this have to do with me, Nina?* Good question. If you happen to be put on a shift with a coworker you don't particularly care for, and you and your coworker are continuously bickering with each other, without trying to get along and accomplish your goals, it could negatively affect both of you. You could be called out by management, moved to another unit, or, worst-case scenario, being "difficult" could lead to you getting fired. Remember what I said earlier? Don't be the reason your boss is stressed! Your employers already have a lot on their plates, and the last thing they want to have to deal with is you and your colleague fighting like children. That looks bad. Very bad. You could be the best certified nursing assistant in the world, but if you're difficult to work with, it will decrease your chances of being promoted. Don't let one rotten apple get you into trouble and ruin your performance review.

Being a Team Player from a Coworker's Perspective

The best way I can describe collaborating with coworkers in the medical field is like having a dance partner. Some will be good, many will be bad, and only a few will ever be extraordinary. You both have your own dance routines to perform, but there are still times when you both have to dance together. Sometimes you have to lead, and other times your partner will lead. Communication plays a huge role when working with other people. You and your colleagues have to be dedicated to doing what is needed from each of you to achieve the same goal. That goal is providing exceptional care to the people entrusted to you.

Remember, you don't have to be best friends with your coworkers, but you do have to keep things civil and professional for everyone's sake. And though I've been focusing a lot on the negatives, you'll find great people to work with and many coworkers may become your second family (since you spend so much time with them) and even friends for life. In fact, I've been really fortunate. There have been so many incredible women and men whom I've worked alongside over the years. These beautiful individuals have helped me become a better version of myself, not only as a caregiver but also as a young woman. I feel truly thankful and blessed to have had them in my life. I wouldn't be where I am today if it weren't for them and everything they taught me as caregivers and compassionate human beings.

Being a CNA is a balancing act between working on your own and working alongside others. When I train new aides, I always tell them to prioritize their patients first. Then, you can go and help your colleagues after. Let's explore why.

If you have ten residents that you're responsible to care for, focus on them first. They're your priority and *you* have specifically been asked to care for *them*. It is their needs that come first. It is your job to give them your undivided attention. If your coworker asks you to help them transfer one of their patients, of course, you should help them. But then continue caring for your own residents. If you know that your coworker is in the middle of caring for a patient, and some of their residents' bells go off, and you're not busy caring for one of your own residents, by all means, you should go and help those patients without having to be asked.

However, keep in mind that there's a difference between helping out your colleagues and being taken advantage of. I've learned this lesson the hard way several times, and you probably will too. Assist your colleagues, but don't do their work for them. The key word being "assist."

An example of this would be that one of your coworker's call bells is ringing. You go and answer it. Their patient needs to go to the bathroom. You assist the patient with walking to the bathroom and tell them when they're finished to ring. You then leave and inform your coworker that you've put Mr. A on the toilet and that he'll ring when he's finished. That is assisting.

What assisting isn't—and what being taken advantage of looks like—is after you put Mr. A on the toilet you're informed by the supervising nurse that you need to give him a shower, get him dressed, and help him shave because they can't find their CNA and Mr. A needs to leave for a doctor's appointment in an hour. Meanwhile, your coworker has been hiding out in the nurses' station, relaxing the entire time or on their phone while all your assigned patient's call bells have been ringing like crazy. True story.

My advice is, yes, help each other out. We are all on the same team and hopefully share the same mission. Don't take advantage of your coworker or employee. Play fair. CNAs, assist your nurses; and nurses assist your aides when they need it. Everyone should be helping each other out for things to work smoothly.

> There's nothing wrong with assisting your coworkers when they need you to, but don't do their job for them. On the same note, don't expect others to do your job either.

The work relationship between nurses and CNAs is both something beautiful and complex at the same time. Do your best as an aide to make sure that you have and maintain a good relationship with your nurse as much as possible. As aides, there are things we can do to help our nurses, such as making sure patients are safe, don't fall, are fed, changed, toileted, and have received a skin moisturizer to keep it intact while doing changes.

The one way that you can achieve being on good terms with your nurse is to communicate like that is your only job. It's better to over-communicate than under communicate information. Communicating can be little things like informing the nurse that Ms. B has been sleeping all day when that's not normal for her. Or that Mr. N said that he's constipated and would like a supplement to help him go to the bathroom. Sometimes it is the smallest pieces of information that can end up being the most critical. Communicating with them clearly helps everyone.

Throughout the years, I've worked with nurses who I've absolutely adored and others who I couldn't stand to work with. Some of it had to do with us having non-compatible personalities, but the main thing that will make or break a work relationship—in my opinion—is the workspace power dynamic.

Whether we like it or not, in healthcare CNAs are seen as the lowest on the totem pole. And although we are nursing assistants, and our job is to assist nurses, some nurses will refuse to have anything to do with patient care. They'll only pass medications, do wound dressings, and take care of documentation. Now I know that nurses have a lot on their plate, but on multiple occasions I've felt as though I was drowning at work because of the amount of patient call bells ringing while the shift nurse was sitting and watching a movie on her phone.

Yes, the responsibility of answering patient call lights primarily falls on the aide who must go into the room, check on the patient, and turn off the call light. But if your CNAs are running around crazily trying to get things done, and the nurse sees there are more call lights than you can manage at that given moment, it would be great if they could lend a hand too. At the end of the day, the patient's well-being is everyone's responsibility, not just the CNAs. Everyone should help each other in patient care.

I once asked a nurse if she could get a cup of water for one of our patients because I was in the middle of giving another resident a shower. She answered that getting a cup of water was below her paid grade and kept on walking. But I've also had nurses tell me they preferred working with me, instead of other CNAs, because their CNAs didn't do their work, or were constantly disappearing when asked to care for patients, or sometimes aides would sit at the nursing station and expect the nurse to do their job for them. None of that's okay. We need to come to a happy medium where nurses and CNAs work well together. And it can be done! My favorite nurse of all times is Linta. Not only because she's a kindhearted human, but because she's an exceptional nurse. She cares for her patients, has a great work ethic, she's efficient, and on top of that, will help the CNAs. She gets the patient's call lights when she can, will help you pull a patient up in bed, and will transfer patients to and from the toilet if needed. When a nurse is willing to help out, it makes all the difference for an aide. That's why I will always help Linta out whenever she needs me to because she always helps me when I need it.

Being a Team Player from a Patient or Family Member's Perspective

When a family brings their loved one to a nursing facility, they aren't told that multiple aides will assist their loved one in a twenty-four-hour period. A family member usually thinks that everyone working at the facility will be available, at any time, to look after their loved ones. You have to be understanding of this, especially when everyone is walking around in the same uniform. To a family member or a newly arrived resident, everyone looks the same and can do any type of work and fill every job position. Think of it like when you enter the grocery store. We sometimes assume every staff member working there knows everything about the store and all its products.

If a new resident, or their family member, asks you for something and you're not caring for that patient that day, kindly introduce yourself first and then explain that you're not their aide that day, but that you'll notify the appropriate person who is so that they can assist them. Now if it's something small, like a resident asking for a glass of water or getting them a snack, get it for them just as long as it coincides with their diet. (Note, if you're not sure, always ask the nurse first what that patient's diet allows for before giving the resident anything.) One request is not going to derail you from your workload, and what matters is that you've shown the family or the resident that you care about them and are listening to their needs. It's the little things that truly matter, and that can improve someone's overall well-being that day.

Now let's address conversation etiquette. I'm going to say this once: **Never speak badly about colleagues you don't like in front of your patients**. It's never okay, and it's unprofessional. More times than I care to remember, I've gone into a resident's room and they inform me of all the facility drama going on that day. "Did you hear that Brittany and Destiny aren't friends anymore? Destiny hooked up with Brittany's ex-boyfriend and now they aren't speaking" is a statement you should never have to hear from a patient. Even if it's true, the patients shouldn't know about it. Don't make your problems your patient's problems as well. I've also had residents tell me before, "Oh, so and so doesn't like you, Nina. They said blah blah blah about you." Again, not cool. Keep that to yourself. It doesn't do you, your patients, or the people you work with any good. Sometimes, it can be hard to keep our thoughts to ourselves, but if you're having a difficult time working with someone, try to work it out among yourselves first. If that intimidates you, consider asking a fellow nurse or supervisor to help mediate the talk. You'll benefit from showing you have a good will to fix things. If things don't get resolved, find the appropriate steps you need to take in your company's business policies.

REAL-LIFE EXPERIENCE

I've worked with a lot of CNAs over the years, but my favorite coworker is Dana. She's the nicest, most hard-working person I know, and one of the most optimistic people I've ever met in my entire life. When we first got paired together, I was a little nervous. I'm not going to lie, I've been a caregiver for over a decade, and Dana was fresh out of CNA school. But to my surprise and delight, she caught on quickly and within weeks it seemed like we had worked together all our lives.

A person can always be taught the basics of caregiving. How to properly transfer someone, how to do an individual's bedtime routine, and how to properly complete a new admission packet. What is harder to teach is how to have a good work ethic and character. Those were two things that Dana innately possessed, so we got on well together. We became such great friends that some of the residents we cared for started referring to us as the "petite-duo" (we are both 5'1"). What matters most though is that we share the same values about what it means to be a certified nursing assistant as well as providing the best quality of care to our patients.

I'll never forget the shift where Dana and I had the worst night ever. Everything that could have gone wrong, did. The unit was a disaster when we arrived. The third aide scheduled to work with us didn't show up, so it was just the two of us for the entire shift with all the residents. And we were getting six new admissions. There were two possible outcomes that evening: sink or swim. We chose to swim. To swim fiercely! How did we achieve this? Correct! By working together. We devised a plan, divided the workload equally, communicated like leaders, and worked together as a **team** of two the entire shift. We cared for all the residents together, including the ones who needed two or more people to assist them. We cared for residents with dementia as well as the new admissions together. The more independent residents who only needed one person to help them, we cared for individually.

By the end of the night, after we had finally gotten the last person into bed, Dana and I sat down for the first time in eight hours. We hadn't eaten dinner or taken our breaks, and we only went to the bathroom once during the entire shift. We were in a daze, amazed at what we had just accomplished together. Dana had been working with her wrist in a brace all night, and my previous back injury, that never healed correctly, had flared up. Moments later, our relief (new shift workers) showed up and her facial expression was of concern. "What happened to you? You look terrible!" Ha! We walked out of work that night in pain and exhausted, but with a great sense of pride. It had been a challenging and difficult night, but none of the residents ever knew it. We had properly cared for them despite the physical pain we were in and despite being short-staffed. The only thing that mattered that night was completing our mission: Providing our patients with exceptional care. We surrendered the "me" for the "we."

PRACTICAL TIPS ON HOW TO BE A TEAM PLAYER

Smooth out disagreements

Try to work out any conflicts your coworkers and you are having before getting management involved in your personal matters. Refrain from gossiping about your colleagues in front of the residents. It doesn't matter how much you don't like each other. It's unprofessional. Be mindful of what comes out of your mouth. You *can* train yourself to do it and you'll be a better person for it.

The patient's well-being always comes first

Prioritize your patients first, but make sure to help out your fellow CNAs and nurses whenever possible. It's good karma, but also, people will remember your kindness.

Go the extra mile

When it comes to assisting residents and their family members, it's the little things that make a big difference in their world. That simple act of kindness will make them, and you, feel great.

Teamwork is your friend

The best way to work with your fellow CNAs when you're on the same shift is to devise a plan. Split the task load equally, communicate, and execute it. What's more, work on the residents that have more challenging situations together and with the more independent individuals separately. This is a great habit to get into and your workload will seem lighter. Change your mindset from a "me" perspective to a "we" perspective.

HELPFUL RESOURCES

"Importance of team management and collaboration in the workplace"
article by Elorus.com

"10 Surefire Tips to Improve Teamwork In The Workplace"
article by Amara Pope

"6 Benefits of Teamwork in the Workplace"
article by Dave Mattson

"Phil Jackson on Teamwork"
YouTube video by CSU Fullerton HCOM

You Are The Team: 6 Simple Ways Teammates Can Go From Good To Great
book by Michael G. Rogers

PERSONAL COMMITMENT

These are the three things I commit to working on
to improve my teamwork:

1. _____

2. _____

3. _____

Date: _____ My Signature: _____

PRINCIPLE 5

PRACTICE EMPATHY EVERYDAY

Being empathetic is not usually something that one can be taught; it's more of something that a person possesses naturally within themselves. I've learned from experience that some people think that being empathetic means they're weak. Other times, people mistake empathy for sympathy, which are two different things. Sophie Huss, Global Director of Talent Acquisition & Training at Arkadin states that "Sympathy means feeling pity or sorrow for someone else's misfortune."

Having empathy instead means "...having the ability to understand and share the feelings of another," says Personal Excellence's Celestine Chua. To state it simply, sympathy is feeling bad for someone else's circumstances, whereas empathy is putting yourself in another person's situation as you try to understand what they're going through and what they're feeling.

It's essential for a CNA to be empathetic. In business, they say you have to know your "WHY" in order to be successful. It doesn't matter how you get there, but you have to know *why* you started your business in the first place. Your "WHY" has to be your guiding reason to get you through the tough times. If your "WHY" for starting your own company is to get rich quick, please your parents, or to become famous, those reasons alone probably won't sustain you when things go haywire. For most of us, if we're struggling to make payroll, you just got dumped, or you didn't get a good night's rest, that's too bad. You still have to get up because you have to make a living to support you and your family. When issues like these arise (and they will), you need a strong "WHY" to keep you going strong day in and day out.

Your "WHY" motivates you to keep going and not give up. It's like when an entrepreneur starts their own company because they identified a problem and then created a solution to fix it. The same thing applies when it comes to being a CNA. You have to know and remember your "WHY."

Try this now and ask yourself, why did you become a certified nursing assistant? Now pause and take that information in for a few seconds.

Let's be honest, if you're looking to get rich, become famous, or both, you're in the wrong industry. A lot of times as an aide, you'll feel as though you're overworked, underpaid, and underappreciated, so it's paramount during those difficult times—and you'll have them—to know your "WHY." Usually, our reason is an emotional one, which takes us straight to *empathy*. You became a CNA because you have a passion for helping others. Maybe your mother was an aide and you saw how many people she brought joy to, so you want to follow in her footsteps. Maybe you just quit your job, are in a career transition, and thought that it would be better than going into retail. Maybe college is not something that interests you, but a vocational school does and seems more accessible. Maybe you want to become a nurse, or a doctor, or a facility administrator and you need to start somewhere. Whatever the reason is for you wanting to be a certified nursing assistant, it's that reason that will guide you throughout your career.

"Learning to stand in somebody else's shoes, to see through their eyes, that's how peace begins. And it's up to you to make that happen. Empathy is a quality of character that can change the world."

BARACK OBAMA

HOW HAVING EMPATHY HELPS/AFFECTS OTHERS

Having Empathy from Management's Perspective

When a company needs to hire a CNA, they look for individuals who can not only perform the requirements of the job but also consider the person's temperament. I've repeatedly seen people who were good aides lose their jobs simply because of their demeanor. Management doesn't want to constantly hear you complaining or see that you're usually in a bad mood. This is something you need to be aware of. When you're on the clock or on break you're a reflection of the company you work for. If you're always being rude to the kitchen staff, patients, or your colleagues don't think that your behavior won't go unnoticed. Your boss might not personally witness it, but trust me, if it goes on for long enough it will definitely get back to your supervisor one way or another.

Now I know that everyone has bad days, even sometimes bad weeks, but if you're always picking fights with your coworkers or if your name is often mentioned negatively and the majority of the residents don't have anything positive to say about you, that isn't good. You want to be a positive asset in your organization, not a negative one. You can be the CNA everyone loves working with! Remember, management sees, hears, and takes note of the best performing employees. Keep a clean record so that the next time a raise, promotion, or bonus is available, your name is considered.

Lastly, another way of showing empathy is to try as much as you can to thank and give encouraging feedback to your bosses. It's not easy being in a management position so remember to be empathetic toward your employers and show them grace too.

Having Empathy from a Coworker's Perspective

When we show others kindness and empathy it's like a cold. It's contagious! Try to think back to a time when someone showed you kindness. For me, I specifically remember being at work one day and it was super busy. Like the kind of night that you want to cry because you're so overwhelmed. That was me. I was running the entire night trying to get all my work completed so that I could give my last resident, who required some extra care, a shower. By the end of the night, when I finally got to them, I was exhausted. When I entered their room, my patient was lying in bed watching TV. I told them I was ready to give them a shower. They replied that they had already taken one. I was confused. They told me that someone else had helped them take their shower. To be honest, I thought they were pulling my leg or were just trying to avoid taking a shower, but I wasn't about to argue with them at 9:30 pm. I was too tired! As I was coming out of the resident's room, my coworker passed by and informed me that she had given my patient their shower, got them dressed, and put them to bed because she had some extra time. At that moment I was so grateful that I almost burst into tears! She had seen me struggling all night and decided to help me out without me even asking her to. The following day I bought her dinner as a thank you.

It's the little things that can make all the difference in the lives of others around you. Try to think of empathetic acts of kindness that you can do throughout the day for others while you're at work like,

- Compliment your coworker on their positive demeanor, styles, scrubs, or great work ethic

- When going to refill your water bottle, ask your colleagues if they'd like water as well

- If you do a coffee run on your break, ask your coworkers if they'd like anything

- Help your colleagues answer their call bells without needing to be asked

- Always say Hello and Goodbye to the people you work with. It's respectful and tells them, "I see you"

- Smile! That smile might be the only good thing your coworker or patient experiences that day

Having Empathy from a Resident
or Family Member's Perspective

I understand how challenging it can be to work in an industry where you're assisting people, especially ones who are ill or are recovering from an injury. But I've learned that it can also be extremely rewarding. Let me tell you a story of a patient that I cared for and whom I'll never forget.

When this person first entered the facility, he made it a point to tell every staff member who entered his room how much he disliked them and how incompetent he thought we all were. I hoped that within a few days he would warm up to the staff members, but unfortunately his less than charming attitude lasted for weeks. I dreaded going into this resident's room every time his call bell went off.

One evening when I entered the gentleman's room to check on him to see if he was all right, he was very rude to me, and I left work that night in tears. The next day I avoided the resident at all costs. I'd almost gotten through an entire shift without having to deal with him when his call bell rang an hour before I was done for the evening. I reluctantly went into his room to see what he needed. All the lights were off, and he was lying in bed. I asked how I could help him, and he requested some medicine, so I turned off his call bell, and I left his room as quickly as I could before he started barking at me.

A few moments later, I went back into his room to let him know that the nurse was with another resident but would be right in as soon as she was done. He didn't respond, but I could hear that he was crying. I asked him if he was okay, and he broke down. He told me that for the last four years he had been his wife's sole caregiver. After years of caring for his wife who was ill, it had become too much for him to manage, and he had to place her in a nursing home due to her worsening condition. He went to visit her every day but now he couldn't. He had gotten injured while doing home improvements and was now stuck at our facility. It troubled him that he had to listen to and rely on "kids" (like me) to take care of him. "I just want to get out of here and see my wife," he said as he wept. I stood in the darkness, stunned and silent. I didn't know what to do or how to help him. Just then, the nurse walked in to give the man his pills. I left his room feeling shocked and saddened, and at that moment I felt his pain. It was an emotionally hard, eye-opening experience.

Up until then, I had thought that this gentleman was mean and heartless, but in reality he was in distress. He missed his wife and took his anger and sadness out on my colleagues and me. He was frustrated and in pain. I felt sorry for him, which is something I never thought could be possible. The following day I found out that his favorite dessert was ice cream. From that day forward, every shift that I worked, I made sure that I brought him a cup of ice cream every night at dinner. By the time he left our facility, we were pals, and it was difficult to say goodbye and see him leave. His last words to me were all thanks and gratitude for the kindness I displayed toward him and how I got him ice cream every night. I'll never forget that man. He doesn't know it, but the three greatest lessons he taught me are:

1. Being empathetic can help you and your resident get along better

2. Being empathetic will always help you help your resident cope through a difficult time and have a good relationship

3. Ice cream really does make everything better!

REAL-LIFE EXPERIENCE

From a young age I've always considered myself to be somewhat of an empathic person, but nothing could have prepared me for COVID-19. I've never felt so emotionally and physically drained before. Some days all I want to do is cry, other times I want to scream, and many days, I just feel numb. I've almost quit being a CNA on several occasions since the pandemic started, but what has gotten me through it is knowing that this isn't about *me*. I have to stay for the residents. So many of them are scared, isolated from loved ones and the world, and many of them are ill. I have to stay strong not only for my own family but for the patients I care for. No matter how challenging it may be at times, I stick it out. I know deep inside all of this is going to make me a better, stronger, and more resilient person.

This past year I've gotten better at listening without responding. Normally this is something that's usually hard for me to do because I love to talk! So many times while I'm caring for a resident, they'll confide in me about a difficult situation they're going through. Sometimes I respond, but now, a lot of the time, I just listen and am present. I've earned my patients' trust, and they like to tell me about their hopes, dreams, and regrets. On the days when I'm feeling sorry for myself, I think of my patients and remember all of the hardships they're going through. I'm the one with the freedom to go anywhere, the one in good health, and the one with a supportive family and a good job!

Can you imagine being stuck in a room by yourself twenty-four hours a day for weeks at a time? Sometimes even more? Being taken care of by a group of strangers, while being physically at your most vulnerable, and not being able to see your family or friends except through a window or a phone screen? Not being able to carry out your daily routine? And not having the little things that surround you at home that bring you comfort? I can't even begin to fathom not being allowed to hold, hug, or kiss my loved ones. When my shift is done, I'm one of the lucky ones who gets to go home and see their family. The residents I care for, instead, can't leave. That's the reason why I stay. I need these residents to know I care about them and their well-being. I've committed to looking after my patients at this time while their families are unable to. I can't let them down. Supporting and improving their quality of life is my mission.

PRACTICAL TIPS ON HOW TO DEVELOP EMPATHY

Put yourself in another person's place

Try to understand and feel how they must be feeling. Or better yet, imagine how you would feel if the same situation happened to you or someone whom you loved. Being empathetic doesn't happen overnight. You need to give yourself a few minutes to clear your head and truly feel what the other person is going through. Gift yourself a moment to put yourself in the shoes of someone else.

Befriend others who don't think, look, love, worship, or vote like you

Surrounding yourself with a diverse group of people will make you more inclined to be empathetic toward others around you. Now remember, just because you're friends or associate with other people who have the same beliefs as you do, that doesn't mean that you'll always agree with everything that they do or say. And that's okay. You can still learn from them and have great experiences. It's crucial to be around others who live differently than you do. It forces you to evolve and grow and see life from where they stand.

> *"A comfort zone is a beautiful place,*
> *but nothing ever grows there."*
>
> AUTHOR UNKNOWN

Love yourself

You have to truly love and accept yourself as you are. If you do, you'll learn to love and accept others as they are, wholeheartedly, too.

Take action

Make a conscious effort to educate yourself daily on new topics that affect your community, your city, your country, even the world. The first time I went to Paris by myself I spent the months before learning everything that I could about France and the Parisian culture before even stepping foot in that country. Learning and understanding how other people and cultures do things is beneficial. It's mindful. We all come from different walks of life. It's a beautiful thing because we have so much to learn and enjoy from each other.

Check your biases

Since the beginning of time, everyone has formed pre-existing gener-alizations about others because we are all raised by different types of families, in different societies, with different histories and ways of life. It's crucial to be aware of that. Having a judgment about something is part of being human and how we are raised. However, that doesn't mean we are "in the right" or that how we think is how things should be. Don't judge a book by its cover. Get to know a person first before creating an opinion about them.

Treat others the way that you would want to be treated!

HELPFUL RESOURCES

"Empathy Is to Great Employee-Boss Relationships"
article by Steve Farber for Inc.com

"Empathy at Work—Why it (Really) Matters"
article by Jacqueline McElhone

"The Importance of Empathy"
article by Julie Fuimano

*Empathy: Discover the Power of Empathy
and How to be More Empathetic to Improve and Empower Your Life*
book by Miranda Dalmasso

"Daniel Goleman on the Three Kinds of Empathy"
YouTube video SuperSoul Sunday by Oprah Winfrey Network

PERSONAL COMMITMENT

These are the three things I commit to working on
to become more empathetic:

1. _____

2. _____

3. _____

Date: _____ My Signature: _____

PRINCIPLE 6

MASTER TIME MANAGEMENT

The one thing that will set you apart from being just an okay CNA to an exceptional CNA is your ability to manage your time efficiently. The definition of time management from Oxford Languages is "the ability to use one's time effectively or productively, especially at work."

When I first became a certified nursing assistant, time management is something that I struggled with. I had a really difficult time learning how to take care of more than one person at a time. I always felt rushed or like I was falling behind on my tasks. I felt that I spent my time playing catch up and this made me super anxious. The loud obnoxious patient call lights ringing every ten minutes only made matters worse. Time just seemed to vanish before my eyes and the patients took their frustrations out on me. Every time I entered a resident's room, I felt like I was in trouble for one thing or another. I had always forgotten something (again), or I was being yelled at by a resident for not providing them with care fast enough.

I had major emotional breakdowns in my car, on my commute back home. Knowing that I had given it 110%, but still having people get mad at me, even though I was trying my hardest, was extremely challenging for me.

Things were rough when I first started working as an aide. That's why I decided to write this book and tell you all of this. It's not to whine or try to make you feel sorry for me, it's so that you can learn from my mistakes so that you don't have to make them. I had to work long and hard to improve my time management skills, and I had to be self-critical, but after a lot of practice and commitment to changing or adjusting some of my behaviors, things at work improved significantly. If I can give you one piece of advice that will boost your work performance overall, it would be to focus on improving your time management skills. Not only will you be able to get things done in the time you have, but it will also reduce your levels of stress.

*"A plan is **what**, a schedule is **when**.*
It takes both a plan and a schedule to get things done."

PETER TURLA

HOW TIME MANAGEMENT AFFECTS OTHERS

Time Management from Management's Perspective

If you want to get promoted, become a manager, or make more money, this is for you. The most basic thing that you can bring to a facility or a company is value. *Why is that?* you might be asking yourself. When you have good time management skills it enables you to be more efficient and productive at work, which in turn will make you a positive asset to your boss and therefore your company too. When your boss is meeting their goals and the company is doing well you will also do well. To be successful as a CNA you must bring value to your facility.

That translates into dollar signs as well. The bottom line is always going to be how much revenue your employer is generating. Is their company making money or losing money? This is very important to understand. Sorry to break it to you, but honestly, your employer doesn't care about your new relationship or that you overslept for the third time this month. Managers are continually looking for ways that they can save and make more money for the company. *Cool, Nina. That's their job. Why should I worry about this?* Well, this is where you come in. You're either going to be part of the reason why your employer is making money or a reason they're losing it. When you show up to work late all the time, are on your phone when you're supposed to be working, or when you don't provide your patients with quality care, all of these things will negatively affect your company's bottom line. Like I said before: Make yourself an invaluable asset to a company or your employer. The easiest and fastest way to achieve that is by improving your time management skills.

> *"Time is money; continually look for ways*
> *to do things faster and better."*
>
> BRIAN TRACY

Time Management from a Coworker's Perspective

Let's cut right to the chase. If you want to waste your own time, that's your choice, but it's not fair to your colleagues to squander their time. Your lack of time management is going to negatively affect your ability to work as part of a team. At any given moment during your shift, there might be several different situations going on. That's why it's necessary to prioritize your time so that it doesn't negatively affect your coworker's performance either. What I mean by this is that you have to plan your work schedule by what not only works best for you, but what works for your coworkers as well. Here is an example: Never take your meal break at the beginning of a shift, during change-of-shift, right before/during/when patient's meal trays arrive, and at the end of your shift. Why? Because when you do it leaves your coworkers short one person at one of the busiest times of a shift. It doesn't matter how hungry you may be, it's simply inconsiderate. That's why most places have certain times staff members are and aren't allowed to take their breaks.

This also goes for the amount of time a break is allotted for. Most facilities allow a thirty-to-forty-five-minute break. Be aware and prepared at all times.

One thing that I like to do that saves a lot of time and energy is setting up my patients at the beginning of every shift. Here is how I set up/prepare for a shift when I just get to work:

First, I gather/restock all the laundry supplies I need for the evening:

- Gowns
- Washcloths
- Hand towels

- Bath towels
- Bed linens
- Bed protective pads

Second, I gather/restock all patient care supplies I'll need for the evening:

- Skin protective lotions
- Pull-ups/ Incontinence pads
- Briefs
- Nonskid socks

Third, I tidy up the nurse's station:

- Sanitize all the counters, desktops, chairs
- Restock the paper cups, lids, stirrers, straws, and snacks

Fourth, I set up my patient's rooms (see steps below)

Lastly, I check on / provide care to ALL my patients.

This is the most critical step of all. Check on all your patients within the first hour of starting your shift!

Setting up Your Patient's Room

Step 1. Bring Supplies into EACH Patient's Bathroom & Set Up Their Bathrooms

Always bring in a full set of bed linens (just in case).

Some patients will have a scheduled shower/bed bath for that day (you'll typically give one to two showers per shift.) Sometimes you won't have to if your patients choose not to shower that day or if the room is empty. Sometimes you might have to give an extra shower that wasn't scheduled because a resident has had an unforeseen circumstance that requires them to be washed. Therefore, always bring with you:

- Large towels (If a patient has a scheduled shower/bed bath that day, you'll need three or four towels)

- Protective bed pad

- Hospital gown

- Hand towel

- Washcloth/wipes (If the patient is incontinent bring in two to three washcloths for toileting)

- Briefs (If the patient is incontinent)

- Pull-ups (If the patient is continent)

- Nonskid socks (If the patient has a scheduled shower/ bed bath that day or if a patient is new)

- Skin rash prevention lotion (used for incontinent patients to prevent skin irritation)

- Body lotion should be used on all patients to help maintain their skin health (unless they refuse it.) Remember, moisturizing reduces skin problems.

- Triple bag each patient's trash can bin in their bathroom (one bag is for trash, the second bag is for soiled linens, and the third bag is set up for the following shift.) Always make sure that each patient's bathroom trash can bin has bags in it. This simple act will be a lifesaver when you toilet/change your patients. It will ensure that your patient's bathrooms look tidy, and it's a time-effective strategy. Keep your patient's bathrooms clean and tidy at all times! Don't leave any soiled clothing hanging up, soiled linens laying on the countertops, or soiled briefs or pull-ups in the trash.

Step 2 Check on your patients/toilet and dress them:

- Knock on the patient's door BEFORE entering their room.

- Enter, say Hello, and introduce yourself. State your job position and the hours you'll be working that day for them.

- Ask if they need to go to the bathroom. (If so, either walk or wheel each patient to the bathroom if they're able to get out of the bed.)

- If a patient is unable to get out of the bed or is incontinent, check their brief to see if they need to be changed. If your patient has voided or had a bowel movement, change them immediately and use the skin irritation prevention lotion.

- Change clothing or the hospital gown of a patient if they've soiled or have spilled something onto their clothing.

- Bring your patients fresh water (check with your nurse to see what the patient's fluid diets are, which patients are on fluid restrictions, and who cannot receive any fluids because they're receiving fluids by IV). **This is very IMPORTANT!**

- Make sure that each patient's room is tidy: Clothes are put away, the bed is made if the patient is out of the bed, and sheets on the bed are clean.

- Make sure every patient's tray table is tidy and clean. No strains or crumbs; throw away old food or empty cups and place all remaining items on the table to one side. That way when dinner comes you can easily place a patient's meal tray onto their table. This simple act will save you a lot of time!

Things can change at the drop of a hat when you work in the caregiving industry. That's why it is crucial to set up your patients in advance. It is going to save you and your patients a lot of time and stress in the long run. Here is an example of why it is crucial to set up your patients at the beginning of your shift. One time at work, my nurse informed me that in fifteen minutes, she needed my assistance with changing a resident's dressing. Even though I had planned on giving one of my patients their shower in fifteen minutes, I had to adjust my time schedule because my nurse's request took priority. Remember, we are certified nursing assistants. So, the resident's shower got pushed back.

I assumed that the dressing change would take only a few minutes, but instead, it ended up taking a lot longer than I had anticipated due to unforeseen medical complications. This set me back in my schedule by twenty-five minutes. I know that this doesn't seem like much, but I had eleven patients to care for that night and had only provided complete care to four of them. Not to mention that I had a resident who was waiting for me to give them a shower and another patient to give a bed bath too. Right after I had finished helping my nurse out, I gave my first patient their shower a half an hour later than what I had originally told them that I would. The resident was understanding of the circumstance thankfully.

An hour later, my coworker (remember, we are team players!) received a new patient, an admission that was proving to be more challenging than expected, so they asked for my help. At that moment, I was getting ready to give my second shower of the night. One of my patients had a bed bath scheduled (as you know, bed baths are quite time consuming and no small feat), but once again, I had to shift my schedule to help my coworker. At that moment, her situation was more critical than mine, and she needed my assistance. What I thought would take no longer than ten minutes ended up taking forty-five minutes. By the time I finally was able to give my second patient their bed bath it was an hour late and this time the resident was not so understanding.

What I'm trying to show with these examples is that you have to be mindful of your time but also flexible with it because things are always changing and evolving. When your colleague needs your assistance, you must be available to help them while still completing your own task load as well.

Time Management from a Patient's or Family Member's Perspective

When it comes to being a CNA, you need to be aware of your patient's schedules. Some residents will want to be cared for early on in your shift, while others will prefer to be cared for last, and those requests are perfectly valid. If you manage your time accordingly, you'll be able to provide quality care to all of your patients.

There will be times when three residents want to get ready all at the same time, so you have to know who is going to take the longest amount of time to care for and who will take the least amount of time to care for. I've had to take care of three or more people at the same exact time on numerous occasions and let me tell you, it isn't easy! But it is doable if you prioritize your time properly. If you're not sure where to start first, ask yourself these questions:

1. Which patients are more prone to have a fall?

2. Which residents are incontinent?

3. Do any of my residents have dementia? (If a person has dementia, they're more at risk of being confused or falling than your other patients)

4. Which residents are my extensive transfers? (A person who is an extensive transfer means that they need two or more people to transfer them to and from a place. If a person cannot put any pressure on their legs or is too heavy for just one aide to transfer on their own, a sit-to-stand lift or a Hoyer lift might be needed in order to do it safely.) But with an extensive transfer, you always need to have a minimum of two people to assist the patient. Start with these patients first and then care for your independent residents after.

REAL-LIFE EXPERIENCES

I once cared for a patient who insisted on getting into bed at 6:30 pm every single night. She expected you to enter her room every night at precisely 6:30 pm to assist her in getting ready for bed, and by 7:00 pm she needed to be *in* bed so that she could watch *Jeopardy!* before she went to sleep. I quickly learned that Ms. P wasn't flexible with her schedule at all. One evening, I was in another patient's room helping them to get ready for bed when Ms. P's daughter burst into the patient's room. She began demanding that I stop caring for the patient and attend to her mother immediately. I firmly, but professionally, instructed the daughter to leave (she had entered someone else's private room without permission) and explained that I would go into her mother's room next, just as soon as I was finished caring for the resident I was in the midst of helping.

When I entered Ms. P's room fifteen minutes later, my supervisor (the nurse), Ms. P, and her daughter were all in there waiting for me. You could have cut the tension in the room with a knife. Ms. P was crying, her daughter was furious, and my nurse looked stressed. The next day I got called into the director of nursing's office. She informed me that she had received a lengthy email of outrage from Ms. P's daughter in regard to the incident. I was informed that from then on, Ms. P's bedtime was to be at 6:30 pm sharp, no exceptions. After that night, I made sure to prioritize my time around Ms. P's bedtime schedule so I would never be late getting her ready for bed. I didn't want to go through that ordeal ever again! All it took was a small adjustment to my own work schedule, and everyone was happy. Sometimes you have to make small concessions, even if it's not ideal. Remember, it's not about you. It's about caring for other people, keeping the peace, and being a team player. Think of the bigger picture.

PRACTICAL TIPS ON HOW TO IMPROVE YOUR TIME MANAGEMENT SKILLS

Get status reports.

The first thing I do every day before I start my shift, is I get a status report. This is a verbal briefing from the previous person who worked on that assignment. They inform the new aide who is relieving them of how each resident was that day. Which patients are incontinent, which are a two or more-person transfer, who is on a special diet or on fluid restriction, who is at risk of falling, and which patients are affected by dementia. All of this should be relayed in a report regarding each patient.

Stock your unit.

The second thing I do is go downstairs and get a full linen cart. Next, I restock all the briefs (or Depends) so they're easily accessible, and then I disinfect the entire nursing station with cleaning wipes. Lastly, I restock the disposable cups, straws, and lids so that we are set up for the night. This takes up the first thirty minutes of my night. By doing this simple step I know that I won't run out of supplies during my shift.

Set up your rooms. Check on your patients.

Next, I make my rounds and go into each of my patient's rooms to check on them. I greet them, see how they're doing, and while I'm in there, I set up their rooms. What does this mean? I bring in gowns, briefs/Depends, linens, creams, and a fresh cup of water to residents whose diets allow it. I also bring shower supplies for those who have a scheduled shower in the evening. Remember to triple bag all the trash cans so that it is easier to remove and dispose of trash/soiled linens. Also, tidy up your patient's rooms so their personal spaces look presentable. If you do this, it's going to save you an enormous amount of time, but more so, it makes residents feel good, clean, and taken care of, which in turn means they feel safe and cared for in your company.

What's more, if you set up your rooms at the beginning of your shift, when things become fast-paced, you'll be ahead of the game. I can't tell you how many times I've observed coworkers starting their shifts and waiting for residents to ring their call bells before going in to check on them. To this day, it blows my mind. You should NEVER do this. "Waiting for things to happen" to then act on them is a bad habit to get into, it wastes a lot of your valuable time, and can lead to a resident getting injured.

Toilet your residents.

After that, I change or toilet each one of my patients. This is crucial. Whether the resident is incontinent or continent, is bed-bound, is a one-assist, or can sit on the toilet on their own, I still ask if they'd like to be changed. Now, be mindful that sometimes patients with incontinence or patients with dementia can't tell if they've soiled themselves or not, so be aware they may display "other signs" like being fidgety, they might tug on their clothes, they might become agitated if they're soiled, or touch their genital area if they're uncomfortable because they're wet. I highly suggest that if you have a doubt, that you check them (let them know first what you're going to do; it's common courtesy, even if they can't fully comprehend you). I learned this the hard way. Once I asked a resident if they were "dry," and they said yes, so I left it at that. The next thing I know, an hour later, I had to do an entire bed change. This not only wastes a lot of time, but it can be harmful to your patients, especially your incontinent residents or those affected by dementia. Not changing or toileting your residents can cause infections such as UTIs (urinary tract infections), skin breakdown, and hospitalization. Never delay taking your residents to the bathroom or changing them if they're soiled.

Anticipate your patient's needs.

Learn what your patient's likes and dislikes are. Here is an example: When I pass out water to my residents, I know who likes ice and who doesn't like ice. Some people will only drink soda, and others will only drink iced tea. The same things goes for meals. Once I had a petite patient who had lost a significant amount of weight in a short amount of time, and no one could figure out why. Well, it turned out that the resident only liked grilled cheese, but none of their meals were that, so the patient had just stopped eating. When the staff realized he refused to eat other food, they began preparing grilled cheese sandwiches for him every meal, and in no time, he gained back all of his weight. If you're still not sure about something just ask.

The same thing goes for temperature. Is a person always hot or cold? Temperature can really affect a patient's well-being *and* mood. I can't tell you the number of times residents will ask me if I'm a mind reader because they were cold and wished that they had something to warm up with. A few moments later, I walked into their room with a blanket and a cup of warm tea. It's all about observation, my friend. If you get good at this, it will save you a great deal of time in the long haul, but more so, show your patients you do care about their needs.

Multitask.

If you're not good at this, oh well, you need to get good at it, and fast. There is no way around it. There are some nights when I'm getting five people ready for bed all at the same time. This is precisely the reason why I set up your rooms ahead of time, for the occasions when everyone's bell rings at the same time, and you have to hit the floor running. After dinner is usually when your patients all want to get ready for bed, so I'll assist one person to the bathroom, then go to the next room and do the same, and so on and so forth. Then I go back to the first patient's room and get them dressed and set up at the sink so that they can brush their teeth. Then I do the same routine with the other residents. By the time I get done with the fifth person, the first person is ringing. So, I go back into their room and get them safely into bed and say good night. The pattern continues until everyone is dressed and in bed for the night.

Eliminate safety hazards.

Keeping your residents and yourself safe should be your number one priority! Do everything you can to prevent or limit any injuries and falls.

Residents who are at risk of falling and patients with dementia will always be your most vulnerable. If they're in their rooms in bed, make sure the beds are as far down to the ground as they can go, or the side rails are up. And always make sure their alarms are ON.

If the resident uses a wheelchair and they're stationary, make sure the chair's brakes are locked. If you need to go to another room to care for a patient, have them stay in their wheelchair at the nursing station if necessary so someone can keep an eye on them while you're away.

Make sure your resident's clothes fit well and aren't dragging where they could trip.

Doorways and hallways should be clear of obstacles so your resident, their wheelchair, or both of you can get through at all times (but especially in case of an emergency).

As a CNA, you should wear close-toed shoes, keep your nails short, and not wear any jewelry that could get caught on or be pulled by anything or anybody. We'll talk more about this in Chapter 8, "Dress Professionally."

HELPFUL RESOURCES

"How to Be On Time Every Time"
article by Dustin Wax from Lifehack

"The Importance of Being on Time for Work"
article by Ruth Mayhew

"3 Reasons Why Punctuality Will Help your Career (Time Management)"
article by Jon Rennie

15 Secrets Successful People Know About Time Management
book by Kevin Kruse

"How to Avoid Being Late for School or Work"
YouTube video by Ways to Grow

PERSONAL COMMITMENT

These are the three things I commit to working on
to improve my time management:

1. _____

2. _____

3. _____

Date: _____ My Signature: _____

PRINCIPLE 7

YOUR CHARACTER DEFINES YOU

There are many positive things about working in the healthcare industry, but there are also many things about it that aren't pleasant as well. One of the most useful pieces of advice that I can give you is to *let things go*.

As a caregiving professional, you have to try and not take things too personally. *Ok, that's nice, Nina, but this is my job, why wouldn't I take things personally?* You've asked so many great questions during our time together, so I'll do my very best to answer this one.

I wish someone would have sat me down before I started my first CNA job and told me, "*You're going to have to remind yourself not to take things personally.*" It would have made things a lot easier for me!

Many tears were shed the first year I became an aide because I took everything to heart. Whenever a coworker got upset with me for not being fast enough or a patient yelled at me for something that another CNA didn't do, I felt sick for the rest of the shift. Incidents like that would completely cripple me for the rest of the day. I was so hard on myself all the time, but I had to learn not to let other people's problems get to me. Of course, you should take personal responsibility for things that you do, but that's all that you can do. You can't stress over things that you don't have control over. "Not taking it personally" means "not to be offended or upset by what someone else has said." This can be a challenging thing to master, but it's critical if you're going to work in the healthcare industry. You have to develop thick skin; otherwise, you won't last.

"A successful woman is one who can build a firm foundation with the bricks others have thrown at her."

(SOURCE UNKNOWN)

Now, that's not to say you shouldn't use your voice when there is something that's concerning you or a problem is occurring. But you need to pick and choose your battles and know when it makes sense to speak up about something and when it is best to just stay silent. Many times, the problem at hand is an issue of miscommunication or misunderstanding. Other times the other person may be having a bad day, or some physical ailment, or problems at home. Remember, everyone is going through something. Try to be the person that believes everyone is doing the best they can with what they have at the given moment.

Character is a standard of excellence. It's what you live by and how you conduct yourself in the world. Character defines who you are and if you're able to step up to the occasion or have the wisdom to walk away from it if there is nothing to gain. Having character to me means how you treat yourself and others when no one else is watching. Do you only arrive to work on time on the days that you know your boss will be there or do you show up to work on time regardless of if your boss is there or not?

HOW NOT TAKING THINGS PERSONALLY AFFECTS OTHERS

Not Taking Things Personally from Management's Perspective

When you take things too personally it's mostly going to have a negative effect on your health as a whole and your work performance. Management must be able to count on you, but they can't do that if you're always stressed, burned out, or are on bad terms with everyone in the unit. You have to learn to only focus on yourself and what you *can* control. A lot of times people are going to project their frustrations and anger onto you, and you can either allow it to enter into your personal space or you can choose not to let it affect you. It took me a very long time to learn how to do this (see the practical tips at the end of this chapter). When I did, I became a better CNA. I was more focused, less stressed, and was more productive at work and in my personal life.

We've discussed this before, but management has a lot on its plate. The last thing they want or need is an employee who takes every comment or situation personally and cannot function while at work. What they do need instead is an employee who knows how to manage themselves in difficult situations, who can manage themselves and their attitude—an employee who doesn't need emotional babysitting. The healthcare industry is fast-paced where everything needs to happen *yesterday*. Conduct yourself in a manner so that management, your supervisor, or your colleagues don't have to worry about you and how you take every single thing they say. That doesn't mean you should let them run you over, but it does mean you need to build yourself up to withstand the inevitable heat and deal with it professionally.

When it comes to your boss, try to go easy on them. Remember that being a nursing home administrator can't be easy. They need to have extremely thick skin to deal with all their different and challenging responsibilities on a daily basis. Administrators manage everything from new resident admissions to hiring new employees. They oversee the facility's finances as well as plan and supervise care throughout all departments. They participate in executive and vendor meetings *and* try to keep the shareholders happy. They deal with hundreds of people a day, so they must be able to stay level-headed and focused on the bigger picture: running a business that provides top-quality care to their patients while treating their employees with dignity and respect.

"People will love you. People will hate you.
And none of it will have anything to do with you."

ABRAHAM HICKS TEACHINGS

Not Taking Things Personally from a Coworker's Perspective

Again, the healthcare industry is fast-paced. People's lives are always at stake. Everyone is in a rush and needs things to be done NOW. Although it seems ridiculous, most people will tell you that there is no time for pleasantries. Doctors and nurses will bark orders at you. When I asked a physician friend about this, she explained it this way to me "People will constantly be telling you what to do and everyone is different, so people will want things set up differently. There is always going to be different way of doing a transfer, taking your medicine, or getting a prescription. You have to adapt to everyone else's requests and demands. As a doctor or a nurse, you also don't have time to really sit down and get to know your patients. It is very matter of fact. There is no room to be human sometimes, which is a hard truth to come to terms with."

This has been the hardest lesson I've had to overcome while working as a CNA. I've always been very sensitive and a people pleaser, a perfect recipe for emotional disaster at times. The first week of work after I graduated, I drove home in tears every single night. Someone gave me a dirty look, a resident raised their voice at me, or I made a mistake, and a coworker got mad at me. These are a few examples of simple things that would make me cry. But after a year of this, I finally came to the conclusion that I could do everything right, be the nicest person in the world, and someone would still end up getting mad at me for some reason. Even when I was doing my best. So why was I getting myself all worked up for no reason? Focus on the things that *you can control*. If Mr. Smith is upset with you and calling your supervisor because you didn't get him ice cream at 10:00 pm due to the kitchen being closed, that's not something to lose sleep over. True story, by the way…That was a fun night!

I also want to acknowledge that on many occasions, which now I regret, I've been snappy or rude to coworkers, and at times I didn't get a grip on my emotions, for reasons that had nothing to do with them. I was either "hangry," tired, overworked, or overwhelmed and responded in unacceptable and unprofessional ways. Looking back at those times, I see how my attitude not only didn't help the situation but it also made my coworkers uncomfortable and more distant. Although I always own my shortcomings, and go back and apologize, I realize I should have handled the situation differently. I can't go back in time and change those moments, but I've definitely learned from them and try to react in a more favorable way today. I see those times as "teachable moments."

There will be many instances where you'll feel patients make racist comments and have trouble with your looks, your gender, or even the color of your skin. Remember, the world is changing, and not everyone has the education and upbringing you have. Not everyone was taught compassion and understanding. You can still make a difference in their lives and prove those old stereotypes wrong. Being treated with kindness can change a person's idea about someone. Sometimes you just have to let things go and tell yourself, "I will not stress about things that are out of my control." When I'm stressed or have a lot on my mind, I hum. I know it sounds weird, but it is a simple way that allows me to relieve my stress. It helps me to stay focused and level-headed. Try to find your stress reliever. I've heard some aides tell me that they sing, do breathing exercises, or think of a happy place. If you're ever having a really tough shift, step off of the unit for like twenty minutes and just go outside (I do this myself). There is something powerful about being outside and experiencing the elements of nature or your city.

Not Taking Things Personally from a Patient's or Family Member's Perspective

There are always going to be things that can ruin your day, but it's up to you to choose to move on from them quickly, especially if there is nothing to gain from sitting with that anger and resentment.

One week I came back to work after being off for four days in a row. After I had received the shift report I began setting up my rooms and checking on my patients. When I got to the third or fourth room it was a patient whom I had never met before, so I prepared to introduce myself. I knocked on the door, walked over to the patient, and just as I was about to say "Hello! My name is..." the patient pointed at me and then hollered "That's her! She's the one who did it!" Before I could ask what I'd done, the patient's son burst through the door and ran over to his mom. He began asking her what was wrong and what had happened. She then proceeded to tell her son that I had taken her clothes to the laundry to get washed and ended up losing her favorite shirt. He then began asking me what I had done with his mother's clothing, where I had taken them and demanded that I pay for all the damage I had caused. Just then the nursing supervisor walked in. The patient and her son told her that I had stolen her clothing and wanted to know what the consequences would be for me. I was floored. Just as the nurse was about to ask me if I knew where the patient's clothes were, the day shift aide walked in with a laundry basket full of the woman's clothes. "Here you go Mrs. S, I told you that I would bring back your clothes before I left for the day." Mrs. S and her son looked stunned and became silent. I never received an apology from the lady or her son. The resident just explained that there were so many of us that she couldn't remember who had taken her clothes.

Not everything negative that happens is deliberately done to spite you. Things sometimes happen and there is no reason for allowing them to ruin your day.

Being a CNA with a good demeanor and character can benefit a patient's health and well-being. It can also give their family members peace of mind that their loved one is in good hands. As discussed before, a patient and their family members need to know that you'll rise to the occasion and not let your temper get the best of you when things go sour. Empathy and understanding come into play here. A resident who is disabled, in pain, or going through significant health issues will not always be in the best mood or looking forward to seeing you. Quite the contrary! I think it's safe to say that *nobody* wants to be in a nursing home or a rehab facility of their own will, so don't expect your patients to be Happy-go-lucky. Again, they're doing the best they can with what life has handed them.

REAL-LIFE EXPERIENCE

I once cared for a woman who didn't get dessert with her dinner because they ran out. I tried offering the resident other options, but she wasn't having it. She only wanted pumpkin pie, and nothing else would do. When she came to terms with the fact that there was no pumpkin pie left in the building, she cried for two hours. When she finally stopped crying, she asked for medication. A few moments later, the nurse went into her room to let her know that, for whatever reason, that specific medication had been discontinued by the doctor. The woman ended up throwing a fit and calling the supervisor. Hours later, when I was finally able to calm her down, she asked me what she had done wrong to make everyone hate her. I told her that no one hated her and that, unfortunately, the things that had happened were out of anyone's control. In my eyes, the resident had two options. She could either focus on every-thing that went wrong that night or try to focus on what she could control and have access to. Thankfully, the next day went a lot smoother. I know that at times it can feel as though everyone and everything is against you, but you have to remind yourself to focus on the positive things, the things you actually *can* control.

Throughout my ten-year career as a caregiver, I've been cursed at, had racial slurs hurled at me, been punched, slapped, spit on, my hair pulled, and bitten. Those are all examples of actions I took personally. But there are times in life when you have to stand up for yourself, and these were some of those times. These are behaviors that are unacceptable and must be called out and stopped.

But there have been other times when I've had to choose my battles. One night it just seemed as though all my patients were mad at me for some reason or another. One resident yelled at me because another aide left them on the toilet for twenty minutes. Another patient was mad at me because I gave them water that had ice in it, and someone else threw a glass cup at my head because I didn't come into their room fast enough when they rang. They missed my head, but the cup shattered all over their floor, and I had to spend the next five minutes picking up all the tiny pieces of glass by hand while the resident cursed me out.

That was a bad shift.

That night I realized that I could allow the mean things that others said about me and how they treated me to affect me negatively, or I could *choose* not to let it get to me. I knew that I was an excellent CNA, and whatever was going on with my patients had nothing to do with me. They were just taking their frustrations out on me. I'm not saying that they were right, or it was the right thing to do, but the truth is I couldn't control how they treated me. Instead, what I could control was how I responded to them. Those were the times I chose to bite my tongue and move on.

And when all else fails, LAUGH. Laugh at how crazy things have gotten. Laugh because it is all just too crazy to be true. Laugh because it diffuses the situation and makes everyone feel better. Try to find humor during your darkest hours; it's a good habit to get into so you don't take yourself too seriously.

PRACTICAL TIPS ON HOW TO NOT TAKE THINGS PERSONALLY

- Take a deep breath and count to ten.

- Walk away and try to notice something new about your workplace or a coworker you hadn't noticed before.

- Recite the serenity prayer: *God/Higher Power, grant me the serenity to accept the things I cannot change, the courage to change the things I can, and the wisdom to know the difference.*

- Pray or meditate.

- Remember that it's them and not you.

- Go on a break.

- Eat or drink something.

- Remind yourself that this job allows you to pay for the things you need right now.

HELPFUL RESOURCES

"Physicians can't take things personally. Here are some tips" article by Suneel Dhand, MD

"How to Develop Thick Skin In the Nursing Field" article by CornerStone Medical

"Top 7 Strategies for Working With Patients as a CNA" article by CertifiedNursingAssistant License.org

The Road to Character book by David Brooks

"Don Miguel Ruiz: How to Not Take Things Personally" YouTube video, SuperSoul Sunday by Oprah Winfrey Network

---

PERSONAL COMMITMENT

These are the three things I commit to working on
to improve my character:

1. _____

2. _____

3. _____

Date: _____ My Signature: _____

PRINCIPLE 8

DRESS PROFESSIONALLY

Have you ever heard of the saying, "First impressions are everything"? Well, if you haven't, it's true. People will judge you within seconds of meeting you based solely on what you're wearing and how you look. A person's choice of clothing says everything about them without them even saying a word. From an outfit, we can tell whether a person has low or high self-esteem, where they shop, what's their socioeconomic status, sometimes we can even tell their nationality, sexual orientation, religion, or political stance.

"Dress for Success."

JOHN T. MOLLOY

Molloy's famous seventies quote (which is the title of his book) is still valid. Your choice of clothing relays a powerful message to others. This statement becomes even more relevant when you start your career as a CNA. What you wear tells people a story about *you*. At this moment, you may be rolling your eyes right and asking yourself, *Why is she making such a big deal about this? Who cares what I wear as long as I do a good job? It's not the clothes that matter but the person in them...* And I get it, I hear what you're saying! I used to think the same way... But I quickly learned your appearance really does matter, especially when working in the healthcare industry. Why? Let's explore what your choice of clothing tells others about you.

HOW LOOKING PROFESSIONAL AFFECTS OTHERS

Looking Professional from Management's Perspective

It will always matter to the director of a healthcare facility that all their employees dress and look professional while at work. It's a reflection of your boss, what the company stands for, and how management operates their facility. That's why medical facilities have dress codes in place that must be followed. Some places enforce them strictly, while others are more lenient when it comes to the rules.

The standard clothing that staff members are required to wear in the healthcare industry are "scrubs"—loose-fitting clothing made of durable material. But it all depends on the facility you work at. I've worked at some jobs where employees wore whatever style of scrubs they wanted to, and I've been at facilities where staff had to wear the same-colored scrubs. I've also worked at places where scrubs weren't allowed at all. At that location, the dress code was a pair of black pants, black shoes, and depending on which department you worked in, you were required to wear a specific-colored shirt. Sometimes your employer will provide the uniform while other times you'll have to procure it yourself.

In my personal experience, I prefer working at facilities that have a formal dress code policy in place. It gives me specific guidelines on what to wear, so I don't have to be choosing what clothes to wear every shift. It elevates the appearance of a facility when everyone is dressed the same and gives the place a more professional status. It also makes me feel like I belong to a team, and we all seem equal, regardless of our economic background and what clothes we can afford or not.

If you follow your company's dress code policy, your employer will feel you care about your job.

Looking Professional from a Coworker's Perspective

I've found from my own personal experience that when facilities have a dress code policy in place, it decreases friction, stress, and bullying within the company and among their employees. I recall working at a facility that didn't have a dress code policy in place, and I was not too fond of the drama that resulted from it. Instead of employees focusing on the quality of care they were providing to their patients, coworkers were more focused on trying to "out-dress" each other. Who was wearing the most expensive, newest, and trendiest scrubs was always the hot topic of the day. There was one coworker who usually took the title. Every time that I worked with her, it looked as if she had just stepped off a red carpet with the assistance of a personal stylist. She dressed to perfection: Her hair was always freshly curled, had a full face of makeup on, and fingernails were always salon-done. When we were assigned to the same shift, I noticed that she always had a different set of scrubs on. Which was very impressive considering that just one set of scrubs can cost a pretty penny.

I, however, always looked plain in comparison to my coworker. I wore my hair pulled back into a messy bun, never wore makeup, and I never wore nail polish. I also wore the same outfit every day, because I bought one matching set at a name brand store and it cost me a fortune. You had better believe that I put those scrubs to good use and took care of them! It took me a month to pay that purchase off my credit card. But even with all of that, it didn't faze me. I didn't care what anyone else thought of me because I was there to work. I also didn't care what my coworkers wore, just as long as they did their job. But not everyone felt like me. It seems silly now that I think of it, but do you know there was once a time when there were all-out fights over scrubs? Two coworkers who didn't get along, and who had set themselves up to be unnecessary rivals showed up to work one night both wearing the *same scrubs*! Let's just say that they got into a huge bickering match. They both insisted that the other one change because it looked tacky for them both to be walking around in the same outfit! Neither one conceded and they both ended up in the nurse director's office. That drama got old after a while.

Dressing and looking nice costs money and usually a lot of it. If you haven't already guessed by now, CNAs don't make that much until they're well established, and for some, being able to afford new scrubs can be hard (they aren't cheap). The first time I worked at a facility that didn't have a dress code, I had to go out and buy my own work clothes. From the time when I got certified, all my jobs had always provided our shirts, so I was only responsible for getting black pants and shoes. Up until that point, I had no idea how costly scrubs were.

Remember, the reason scrubs are worn in medical facilities is because they're made to withstand long hours of working, they're stain-resistant, have large pockets, and above all, they're more comfortable to wear than our regular clothes. What's more, they help patients identify who is the staff and who isn't. In big facilities, the color of scrubs distinguishes the doctors, nurses, surgeons, and admins from each other.

When buying a pair of scrubs, it's pertinent to look for premium quality because, first of all, you'll be wearing them all day. Best quality doesn't mean expensive though; it means you need to do your research and find a pair that's going to last a long time, which can withstand getting dirty, and some major hard machine washing. Now you can get scrubs at Walmart, but if you're petite like me, or too tall, you might have some difficulty doing so. I could never find my size, and when I did, they were always too big, so I finally had to give in and buy my scrubs, where all the "popular aides" bought their clothes from—the mall. I was astonished by how expensive everything was! I bought two scrub tops, and a pair of pants, and just those three items alone ended up costing me almost my entire paycheck. Now I only buy quality scrubs. Yes, they're more expensive, but they last longer than cheap scrubs that wear out easily. I've had the same scrubs for a few years now and they're still in great condition. That's why I now factor dress code policy into my decision-making process when considering working for a facility.

Looking Professional from a Patient's or Family Member's Perspective

When facilities require their employees to follow a dress code policy, it not only benefits their staff members but their patients and family members as well. On any given day, a patient might be seen by five to ten different staff members in one day, so remembering everyone's names is nearly impossible. I have trouble remembering my own name some days, so I can't even imagine how difficult it must be for a senior citizen! What I mentioned earlier that scrubs help identify staff, is true. Many patients have told me that when they need something, they know who to ask based on what the individual is wearing. Let me elaborate more on this.

At the facility that I currently work at, everyone wears a different-ent colored button-down polo shirt based on what their job title is. Doctors wear white lab coats, nurses wear red shirts, CNAs wear gray ones, and kitchen employees wear black ones. This is a visual cue to everyone what your position in the company is. Residents have told me that when they need to go to the bathroom, they look for someone who is wearing a gray shirt; if they need medicine they look for a red shirt, and if they want to put their meal order in they look for someone who is wearing a black shirt. It simplifies things for the patients and works very well for the staff too, so they're not receiving requests they can't fulfill. This policy has also benefited me as a CNA because it eliminates awkward moments from occurring when I can't meet a patient's needs.

REAL-LIFE EXPERIENCE

Throughout my years as a certified nursing assistant, I've listened to both sides of why employees are in favor or opposed to wearing a dress code or not. For those of you who are opposed to the idea, I was right along with you when I first became an aide. *I wanted to wear what I wanted to, whenever I wanted to.*

Then, when I found out that at my first workplace as a CNA they had a dress code, I was pretty disappointed, but I learned to live with it. The biggest reason I've found why people are against wearing a uniform to work is because they feel it infringes on their individuality. And that's definitely how I felt! But, I've learned over the years that if you have to wear a uniform, there are plenty of ways that you can add your own personal style to it and still comply with your company's dress code policy. One way that I did this was with my hair.

From the time I was a little girl, I've always loved bright colors. Very bright colors! When I was old enough to start dying my hair, I began getting it braided with bright colors highlighted throughout. In my eyes it was beautiful, and I loved it. I never even thought that this would be a problem. But I quickly found out that while working at a nursing home or rehabilitation facility it was. My boss at the time told me that I wasn't allowed to wear my hair in bright colors. I could only wear my hair in natural colors. With time I noticed that the medical industry is a lot more conservative than other industries, so when it came to working in the field and with patients directly, one on one, I had to figure out how to incorporate my personality in a different way. Also, older generations may feel uncomfortable with colors that are too bright, and you don't want to be making patients feel uneasy or scared around you. In the end, having a job was more important than expressing my personality the way *I wanted* to. I ditched my hot pink braids and found a good compromise: I exchanged them for bright gray braids instead. A few years later, my hair has become my signature look. Well, that and my bright neon sneakers are the first things that patients usually notice about me. I've learned that I can be myself and follow the rules at the same time.

PRACTICAL TIPS ON HOW TO LOOK PROFESSIONAL

When applying for jobs

During an interview always find out if the company you're applying to has a dress code policy or not. If so, find out how formal or informal it is beforehand. Calculate how much you're going to need for clothes and decide to start setting money aside. Some companies may offer clothing, work shoe discounts, or allowances for scrubs as a benefit. Ask if this is something they offer. And if they don't, make the suggestion to HR.

Have a work clothes budget

Set up a savings account that's specific to buying work outfits. Now I'm not talking about a shopping spree. I'm referring to an emergency fund in case anything unexpended happens. If you have a bank account, have a small amount of every paycheck automatically transfer over to a savings account that becomes your emergency fund. Once, at work, I stepped into feces while changing a patient, and my entire sneaker was ruined. RUINED. The next day I had to buy new shoes. It ended up costing me a hundred dollars that I didn't have. Let's just say I learned the hard way. Prepare for emergencies now, so you don't have to be asking family or friends for money to buy *your* work clothes later. Or so you don't have to call out of work because you don't have the appropriate attire to wear for work.

Get the right clothes.

Make sure to buy scrubs that are a size bigger than you are. I'm an extra small, but facilities usually don't carry my size, so I always get stuck wearing a small or medium-sized shirt. I've found this to be a blessing in disguise. I would rather work in clothing that's a bit loose-fitting than tight-fitting clothing. Remember, you'll have to bend, lean, stretch, pull, push, maybe even sit down, so you want a material that gives enough room to do these activities. But don't get them too big, as they could become a safety hazard. You don't want to be tripping over your pant leg or have food falling down your shirt if the neck opening is too big. You just want enough space to move comfortably around. It's also beneficial in cases of weight gain, dryer shrinkage, and pregnancy. There is nothing worse and costly than continuously purchasing new work attire every few months due to unforeseen circumstances.

Your shirts, pants, scrubs, underwear, and shoes should be CLEAN (no stains), and odorless before you start your shift. Make sure that you wear a belt if you have to wear slacks to work. There is nothing worse than mooning your colleagues and patients while at work. It's gross, and nobody wants to look at that. Ladies make sure that your cleavage is covered too.

Wear clean and supportive undergarments. For my female readers, if you haven't done so yet, get fitted for the right bra! Most women buy and wear the wrong kind of bras that don't support their body types, and that can cause major discomfort or back pain. Getting fitted for the right bra is free, and once you know the right kind and size bra you should be wearing, you'll feel much better about yourself and more comfortable.

Lastly, always wear clean socks and closed-toed shoes.

Grooming matters.

When it comes to your hair, wear it out of your face. If you have long hair, put it in a ponytail or a bun. If not, keep it short and manageable. There are so many different and affordable accessories for keeping our hair out of our face these days that there is no excuse for not doing so. Having someone else's bodily fluids or food get in your hair can be pretty gross. Take my word for it! It happened to me once, and when I say that I had a conniption, it isn't an understatement. Also, most facilities will only allow you to wear your hair in natural hair colors such as black, brown, blonde, red, and gray. Pinks, purples, blues, yellows, oranges, and greens aren't usually permitted. Trust me. I've tried.

This next one might get me into trouble, but I'm going to say it anyway. When it comes to wearing makeup at work, I believe that less is more. I know that this is everyone's personal choice, so I'm not going to harp on this topic for too long. I choose not to wear makeup when I go to work. I wore makeup once, and by the end of the night, I looked like I had two black eyes. A smokey eye makeover and a sixteen-hour shift just don't mix well together. I've known coworkers who have come into work wearing pageant makeovers, and they did just fine. So again, it's everyone's personal decision. What I do know is that you're also not going to want to spend the little break time you have fixing your makeup in the bathroom. And you shouldn't be in the bathroom fixing your makeup if you're supposed to be on the floor caring for patients. Use your break time wisely on something else, like getting some fresh air, stretching outdoors, or even indulging in a healthy snack.

Wear natural smelling colognes and perfumes. I used to wear perfume until I worked with a resident who had such a bad reaction to my perfume that it caused them to throw up. Guess who had to clean that up? Remember, it may smell good to you, but it may not smell so nice to others around you. Especially when you're working with infants or individuals who are ill, recovering from a severe injury, have dementia, or are dying. Be mindful of your scent because it may cause a negative physical reaction in someone else.

Speaking of odor. SHOWER. Bed baths don't count! I know that showering is not something that happens on a daily basis in many cultures. However, if you live in the US, you should be able to take a daily shower. Remember, showering removes the dead skin cells from your body, it clears the pores and lets your body breathe through your skin (your skin helps your body eliminate toxins). Showering also removes any bacteria that may cause odor or infections, and a good shower can make you feel great and revitalized or relaxed.

Always carry a travel toothbrush kit in your bag and supplement it with mouthwash or mints. Avoid gum (it just doesn't look good and isn't good for you). Having good-smelling breath is important. Trust me. I'm sure that your patients and coworkers would agree with me on this one!

Nail hygiene. First, make sure they're short and clean, and scrub them often. Bacteria, germs, and a wealth of other gunk can get under your nails and contribute to the spread of some infections.

Here is where I'm going to get in trouble: Fake nails. This rule used to be enforced a lot more strictly, but I've found that over the years it has become a lot more relaxed. I don't wear fake nails for two reasons: One, I'd rather save that money for something else more long-lasting. Two, I find it difficult to do care for my patients while wearing them. I even choose not to wear colored nail polish to work, but when I do, it's clear or a natural shade. Once I had a resident ring me, and when I went into their room, they complained that there was a bug in their food. When I looked closer, I realized that my coworker's long black acrylic nail had come off and fallen into my patient's salad!

A lot of facilities discourage the use of artificial nails, but still, some staff members ignore it. All I have to say is it's your choice, but if you accidentally scratch, point, stab, or cut a patient with your fake or long nails, that's on you, and it could become a serious issue. And you don't want to injure yourself by breaking a nail and then having to miss work because of that. That's simply an embarrassing excuse. There is a time and a place for everything. Long acrylic nails just don't mesh with hands-on caregiving.

The same thing goes for jewelry. Many companies discourage it for safety reasons, but not everyone listens. Keep your jewelry to a minimum. I choose to only wear studded earrings, so they don't get in the way of my work. I've seen colleagues injure themselves—or a patient—because they wore big hoop earrings, bulky rings, or long necklaces. Just avoid the trouble altogether. You can still look great, be you, and be memorable with less!

HELPFUL RESOURCES

"Cracking The Healthcare Dress Code"
article by Danielle Kalberer

"Image Check: Impact Of Employee Appearance On The Patient Experience"
article by Alan A. Ayers

"Medical Office Dress Code Policy"
article by Lorraine J. Floyd

Business Etiquette Made Easy: The Essential Guide to Professional Success
book by Myka Meier

"CNA State Exam Dress Code and Tips"
YouTube video by Legacy Healthcare Careers Nursing Assistant School

PERSONAL COMMITMENT

These are the three things I commit to working on
to improve my professional appearance:

1. _____

2. _____

3. _____

Date: _____ My Signature: _____

PRINCIPLE 9

SELF-EDUCATION CREATES CONFIDENCE AND OPPORTUNITIES

When it comes to working in the healthcare industry, your patients must trust you. The fastest way to build someone's trust in you is by believing in yourself. The fastest way to build confidence within yourself is through continuous education. You're never too young or old to start (or continue) self-educating yourself.

I know what you're thinking: *Nina, that's nice and all, but I already went to CNA school, so I'm good. I know everything I need to get a job now.* I understand what you're saying but hear me out. When I say the word "education," automatically you're probably thinking of going to school, college classes, expensive online webinars. Yes, that's one form of education, but there are several ways that we can become "educated."

The one that I'm referring to is self-education. The definition of self-education is "the act or process of educating oneself by one's *own* efforts especially through informal study" states Merriam-Webster. Think reading, listening to podcasts, journaling, staying up-to-date on current events (pick your news sources carefully!), watch a documentary or docuseries on PBS, or an educational video online. All free activities! Maybe even consider signing up for a class or checking out a book on a topic that you're interested in learning more about (local libraries offer a wealth of free online resources, classes, and materials).

Unfortunately, after you graduate from CNA school, there isn't much continuing education that follows or that you're encouraged to do. So it's up to you to educate yourself to get ahead and improve your quality of life. This is crucial because acquiring more knowledge will help you become a better CNA and become a better human being. Like Rejoice Denhere says, "The most powerful people are the ones who never stop learning."

HOW SELF-EDUCATION AFFECTS OTHERS

Self-Education from Management's Perspective

Having informed and confident certified nursing assistants is key in the healthcare industry. That's why some nursing home directors will provide their staff with additional educational tools and resources to make their employees stronger and more competent. Some companies will pay their employees to go to school to become certified nursing assistants or nursing school, either through a tuition reimbursement benefit or an education assistance program.

Other companies sometimes host healthy living events once a year at their facilities. Which is like a health fair. Speakers come in and do presentations on healthy lifestyle habits that can be implemented into your life to make you feel and function better, such as ways to improve your nutrition and exercise. Also, sometimes companies invite outside instructors to come in and teach a class such as CPR or First Aid Training. This is an excellent way for employers to build self-confidence in their aides so they can provide the best quality of care to their patients. I've experienced firsthand that companies whose facility directors provide educational resources for their staff members are more likely to have higher employee satisfaction rates and better reviews from their residents. This, in turn, results in an increased bottom line, more customers, happier customers, and a great reputation among competitors.

Self-Education from a Coworker's Perspective

Building strong relationships at work and in your industry is essential to advance your career, to connect with people in your trade, and to develop a healthy support system. In other words, you need to create a strong professional network. To become more knowledgeable in your field and a more confident person, you have to surround yourself with other like-minded people.

> *"If you want to go fast, go alone.*
> *If you want to go far, go together."*
>
> AFRICAN PROVERB

The fact of the matter is, that if you want to become a better person, you need others in your life to help and support you as you go through your journey to becoming the best version of yourself. That's why it's crucial to develop a tight-knit group of relationships within your industry or field. Now I know this may seem like something only highly educated individuals do, but everyone should be doing this. Self-education is for everyone; it's not just intended for a few lucky people. You're never too young or old to learn something new, and you may find great joy in learning about things you're passionate about.

You probably won't believe me when I tell you that some of the greatest teachers and mentors I've ever had have been my coworkers. My colleagues have taught me so much over the years, from little, practical, everyday life matters, to actions or physical details that can save someone's life. The wisdom they've given me spans from which grocery stores are the best to buy healthy foods from, to what kind of shoes are the best to wear at work, or what sprays do the trick when getting a child's marker out of your scrubs. These don't seem like much, but they're all valuable things to know that you're probably not going to learn from a textbook. I'm continually discussing new recipes, workouts, and vitamins my coworkers and I should try. You may think that this is ridiculous and has nothing to do with becoming a better CNA, but that's where you're wrong. This has everything to do with improving your quality of life and life skills, which in turn can help you become an exceptional aide.

Having conversations with other people, asking for advice or help in an area you want to know more about is one of the easiest ways to improve your knowledge. This knowledge can help turn your weaknesses into strengths in your life and your career. Like Francis Bacon said, "Knowledge is power." When you self-educate, you create opportunities to increase your self-esteem, skills, and financial income. So never stop learning new things. Allow yourself the opportunity to be better.

Self-Education from a Patient's or Family Member's Perspective

Patients must trust that their CNA knows what they're doing and can provide them with the best care possible. I feel it's really crucial for employees, but especially CNAs to put themselves in their patient's shoes. Try to understand what it's like to be on the other side of things. As an aide, your mission should be to provide your patients with exceptional and quality care.

A lot of patients know that their life and well-being are in *your* hands. I often put myself in their shoes and wonder what it must be like to completely depend on someone to get you out of bed in the morning and dress you. To take you to the bathroom or change your pads. To bring you food when you're hungry or a blanket when you're cold. I empathize wholeheartedly with what it's like to have to constantly have to ask for things to be done for you because you're no longer able to do it yourself.

The way to make a patient feel at ease and safe is for their caregivers to have confidence in themselves. Knowledge creates confidence, and confidence creates trust. Have you ever met someone and just felt that everything would be okay because of how confident the person was? That is very important. There is nothing worse than going to the doctors and feeling as though your physician has no idea what they're doing or what they're prescribing you. I've been in that situation before, and as a patient, I can tell you it's horrifying. You've spent time, money, and energy for someone to help you with something that you cannot do for yourself, and they have no clue what to do. That's why it's essential to always be self-educating yourself. In medicine, there is always new information coming out or being updated. As an aide, it's your responsibility to stay current with all of the latest machine equipment, transfer techniques, and physical therapy tools. Yes, your company should provide for that training too, but don't always wait for it to happen. Be proactive. Demonstrate interest in being more knowledgeable and learning something new. When a person is in a nursing home, in long-term care or assisted-living residence, or even in a rehabilitation facility, the last thing they should have to worry about is that their aid doesn't know how to do their job properly.

REAL-LIFE EXPERIENCE

The greatest life lesson I've discovered within the last few years is the gift of self-education. Depending on which company you work for, some educational materials will be provided to you after you become certified, but unfortunately, there aren't that many dedicated resources out there for CNAs yet. The majority of things that I've learned in my professional career as a CNA have been through hands-on life experience. However, there is a wealth of medical and healthcare knowledge out there for us to continue learning. Libraries are full of free databases with articles, manuals, healthcare studies, medical journals. Find a topic you're interested in and ask for help on getting that information. It's all there for you if you choose to find it. And if you don't know what things mean, ask for help. People who know about a topic are usually happy to share resources and information with others who are passionate about subjects like they are.

When I started working at my first job as a CNA, I felt I had made a terrible mistake. I've always been incredibly shy, so working in a fast-paced and unpredictable environment was scary to me. But thankfully, I didn't give up. I had kind coworkers who came next to me and showed me the ropes. And I had the humility to know it was in my best interest to take their advice and learn (don't get on the defensive!) that what they were teaching me was not to make me feel flawed or inadequate, but because they cared and wanted to make me a better CNA and a more valuable employee. I've also had the gift of making several mistakes throughout my career. Through those many failures, I've learned what *not to do*. Some missteps took longer to figure out than others, but I eventually did. I've grown the most from my failures and have had the most success. That's one of the main reasons I wrote this book—because when I went to school there wasn't a book like this. I want you to be better than me and learn from my mistakes.

During my time as a CNA, I've cared for hundreds of people. All those years of hands-on experience and practice have allowed me to become more confident in myself and in my ability to care for others.

Never stop learning and believing in yourself.

PRACTICAL TIPS ON HOW TO CONTINUE TO SELF-EDUCATE

Your local library

- Get a free library card.

- Ask the librarian where you can find the topics you're interested in. Check out books, audiobooks, magazines, search their medical resources and databases.

- Take an online class (all public libraries offer free continuing education to their patrons) on various topics from personal development to career development.

Your city/neighboring cities

- Take a free emergency response program with your local fire department.

- Get a first aid or CERT (Community Emergency Response Team) training.

- Find an extension program at your local community college.

- Enroll in a class at your local adult school.

- Go to a conference, meet new people, and expand your horizons and your network!

Your company

- Ask if your job offers paid training programs. If it doesn't, ask if they'd consider tuition reimbursement to take a class relevant to your job.

Join local organizations

- Many local organizations offer free classes or workshops for their residents. YMCA and SCORE are very popular with free or affordable classes. SCORE even offers free mentorship opportunities.

Use your phone as a tool

- Listen to podcasts. This is a great activity to do while you're in the car, or out on a walk, or during a bout of insomnia.

- Get on a sleep schedule. Learn how many hours someone like you needs to recover after a hard day of work. Try to commit to it a few days a week. A rested body and mind make all the difference!

- Download a workout program, a fitness tracking app, and even a meditation app.

- Get an app with walking or hiking trails in your city.

- Schedule monthly times where you and your coworkers or friends can get together outside of work to talk, relax, eat, and have fun. If you can't get together in person, do an online video call to check in with each other.

Use your computer as a tool

- Take cooking, yoga, language, computer, or even a business management class.

- On Facebook or LinkedIn, join online groups that are specific for CNAs. You'll never guess the wealth of knowledge that's shared there for free!

- Watch exercise tutorials on YouTube that will strengthen your back, legs, and arms.

- Use social media to follow experts (not influencers!) in areas of your life that you're trying to grow and improve in.

- Take financial literacy classes to manage your finances better. What's more, make a financial plan. It will give you peace of mind and help you reach your goals quicker.

HELPFUL RESOURCES

"How to Educate Yourself and Be an Effective Self-Learner"
article by Leon Ho

"Want to Keep Learning? Look to Your Co-workers for Inspiration"
article by Jeannette Eaton

The Science of Self-Learning
book by Peter Hollins

"How to Build Self Confidence" CeCe Olisa, TEDx Fresno State
YouTube video, TEDx Talks

SCORE Workshops

PERSONAL COMMITMENT

These are the three things I commit to working on
to improve my education:

1. _____

2. _____

3. _____

Date: _____ My Signature: _____

PRINCIPLE 10

THE POWER OF KINDNESS

The most valuable lesson that I've learned throughout my caregiving career has been witnessing and experiencing firsthand the extraordinary power of what treating people with kindness can do. Oxford Languages defines kindness as "the quality of being friendly, generous, and considerate." Being kind is a simple act that can have profound and lasting effects on other people's lives.

"Happiness is the new rich. Inner peace is the new success. Health is the new wealth. Kindness is the new cool."

SYED BALKHI

As humans, we are designed to remember events, people, and things based on our emotions and experiences. Think back to when you were a child. You either remember the kids in your class who were nice to you or those who were mean to you. Often, more times than not, our brains tend to focus on the people, places, or experiences that were unpleasant rather than the pleasant ones. Although I've accomplished so much throughout my life, just one mean word or phrase can take me back to middle school days when I was mercilessly bullied by a classmate.

To this day, I still remember the sound of this kid's voice, the way that my stomach went into knots every time I walked into school, and how no one came to my defense. Not the teachers, my so-called friends at the time, and not the kids who felt badly for me because they knew it was wrong but silently stood by and watched it happen. He changed my name to "Snitch," spoke badly about me to the other kids in our class for hours on end while I was sitting right next to him; once he even pushed me into a locker. Basically, this guy made fun of all my insecurities publicly for the entire year. The fact that my hair was falling out, or was too short, my severe acne, and that I was ugly because I'm dark-skinned. The only place that I could seek solace from his never-ending humiliation and abuse was by hiding out in the bathroom.

The only people who did help me get through that hellhole of a time were the school nurses. Their office became my safe space and I'm truly thankful for the kindness and understanding they showed me. *Well, that's sad and all Nina, we've all been through something, but why should this matter to me?* You might think I want your pity, but no. I'm sharing my story with you because as a CNA you must treat yourself, your boss, your coworkers, and above all, every single patient you care for with kindness and dignity. You don't want someone to be telling a dreadful story like this about you ten years from now. You don't want to be known as the bully, the disrespectful one, the ill-speaking resentful coworker. Even adults get their feelings hurt. And it can still affect your self-esteem no matter how old you are.

Remember, your words and actions carry weight. You might not think anything of what comes out of your mouth, but the people you work with or care for will either be positively affected by your actions and words or negatively affected. There was one day at work that I was particularly stressed because I had a lot going on in my personal life. But I thought that I had hidden my stress pretty well. I had kept it all nice and tucked inside for nobody to see. However, I was wrong.

At some point during my shift, a nurse came out of a patient's room whom I had just cared for. The nurse asked me what I had said to the resident. I was perplexed and told him I hadn't said anything out of the ordinary. The nurse informed me that he had found the resident crying right after I had finished providing care to them. I was shocked. I hadn't done anything! So, hoping to clarify the situation calmly, I went back into the patient's room to find out what was the matter. The patient looked at me and asked, "Why are you mad at me?" I stood in her room, stunned. Her question caught me off guard... I told the resident that I wasn't upset with her. With tears streaming down her cheeks and swollen red eyes, she said, "You aren't acting like yourself today."

I was confused at first, and then it hit me. I understood what she meant and where she was coming from. You see, I was usually laughing, joking around, and very talkative with the woman, but that day I was not. I had kept our conservation very matter fact. It was short and to the point. I was tired, had a lot on my mind, and was not in a good mood. The woman mistook my serious demeanor and quiet manner that day for me being mad at her. At that moment, I was pulled out of the little box I had shut myself into and realized that my words and actions always have an effect on other people, even when I don't intend them to.

I dried the woman's tears, assured her that I wasn't upset with her in the slightest, and I got her two pieces of cake that night as a peace offering. We both felt good after that.

"You can be rich in spirit, kindness, and love and all those things that you can't put a dollar sign on."

DOLLY PARTON.

Being kind doesn't financially cost you a thing. So, to put it simply: BE NICE!

HOW A FRIENDLY DEMEANOR AFFECTS OTHERS

A Friendly Demeanor from Management's Perspective

Having employees who are kind and caring is extremely valuable to your employer. The healthcare industry is a business based on caring for people. They need to employ individuals who are kind and have positive attitudes; otherwise, their company will severely suffer—giving them a bad reputation, a higher employee turnover rate, and, most likely, a financial loss. Management knows this when hiring CNAs to work for their company, but you'd do well to keep it in mind too.

It's a no-brainer that having kind and friendly employees increases team spirit and morale within the workplace. "High morale will allow for better production as when employees feel positive and enjoy their working environment, they'll feel more satisfied and far more moti-vated," states Heather Harper, organizational psychologist, and lead content manager for The Career Project. When you're kind and friendly at work it will create a positive environment and culture at your facility. This could result in you receiving great reviews, which could open doors to better opportunities within a company such as getting promoted and earning more money.

A Friendly Demeanor from a Coworker's Perspective

It's crucial to display a positive demeanor while you're at work. I know that we are all human, so you can't be expected to be happy all the time, but you do need to treat others with respect. That's non-negotiable. Don't take your frustrations out on your colleagues; leave your drama at the door. What does this mean? It means that when you enter work, all the things that are going on in your life outside of work shouldn't affect your work performance or your temperament. Be the coworker who lights up the room with their positive energy, not the one who drains it.

I remember a shift I had that was just a bad night. There were several staff callouts, we got a few admissions that were very challenging, and it was pouring rain outside. The energy in the unit was tense. So, our supervisor bought pizza for the entire floor as a way of saying thank you for all our hard work. We were all so happy. Not because we were going to have pizza (anyone can have pizza), but it was *unexpected*. It was a gesture from a supervisor toward us, which demonstrated many things: "I see you. I've been paying attention. You're all doing a great job. I appreciate you." Just that small act of kindness only positively changed the environment of the wing. All of a sudden everyone was smiling, laughing, and the energy became a lot lighter.

The Quiet Revolution article "6 Science-Backed Ways Being Kind Is Good for Your Health" by Maile Proctor gives some pretty compelling reasons why we should be kind to each other at work.

1. Being kind releases feel-good hormones. It boosts your serotonin levels (the hormone that stabilizes our mood, our feelings of well-being, and happiness). This is also known as "Helper's High"

2. Kindness eases anxiety. Like when someone gives you a compliment. It can make you relax

3. Kindness is good for your heart. It can lower your blood pressure

4. Being kind to others can help you live longer

5. When you smile it can reduce your stress levels and make you feel better. (I recommend that when you're feeling low, watch a funny movie, listen to a funny podcast, or watch a clip of your favorite comedian)

6. Kindness prevents illness. (I suggest you try volunteering. It is good for you, emotionally and physically. Every community needs volunteers, even for the simplest things like reading a book to seniors or delivering books from the library, or food)

Yes, everyone has bad days, even sometimes a bad week, and that's okay and it's human. But you have to be able to compartmentalize it in a way that doesn't affect others. Have you ever worked with someone whose presence sucks up all the positivity in the air? There is nothing worse than working with a negative Nancy or Niles. It's extremely stressful.

For the rest of my life, I'll never forget this one specific coworker even if I tried. They were one of the meanest people I had ever met in my entire life. This woman would get mad about anything and everything. If I asked her for help with a patient, she would flat out refuse, so I had to figure it out on my own. If I asked her if she needed help with anything or anyone, she became angry and hostile. I started avoiding her at all costs, which is hard to do when you're assigned to work with that person on the same shift. Things got so bad that I began having panic attacks before each one of my shifts in my car. Just the thought of having to work with that woman made me feel ill and it was affecting my physical and mental health. The only solution I could find was asking my manager not to pair me up with that aide anymore. When my request was granted, I was overjoyed and relieved. **Don't be that coworker that nobody wants to work with.** And if that's you, then try to ask for help where you need it instead of taking it out on others that support you. There are resources for everything in life. Working in the healthcare industry is already stressful enough without all the employee drama, so again, just **BE NICE** to each other, please. We're all on the same side!

A Friendly Demeanor from a Patient's or Family Member's Perspective

Since the start of my career as a CNA, I've received the same compliment everywhere I've gone: "I like you the best." I've been told this by many patients and their family members, and I'm sharing this here for a reason.

For the longest time, I was appreciative of the acknowledgment but didn't think anything of it. Eventually, I began asking some of these residents why they preferred that I care for them instead of other CNAs. At the end of the day, we had all studied to get certified as nursing assistants and had all been interviewed by the same company we were working for. But why did they prefer me instead of others if we had all been trained the same way? One man responded, "Because you're the nicest, kindest, and sweetest one here." At that moment, it dawned on me. **There could be two people who are equally qualified in skill, but if one person is kind and the other person is indifferent, people are going to naturally gravitate more toward the nicer individual.**

The reason I'm saying this is because in healthcare, it's crucial to listen to those you're caring for. My business mentor, Gary, tells me all the time that companies should be listening to their customers more and act on the feedback they receive, whether it's good or bad. If you don't, then even if you have a business, it most likely won't be successful. The same is true when it comes to healthcare. The most common complaint, negative feedback, or concern that I've heard throughout the years from residents and their families have all been in regard to being treated *unkindly* by staff members. When I say "unkind," I'm not referring to abuse. There is a very clear distinction. Being unkind is something else.

Let's say you're at your local grocery store, and you're getting ready to get in line to check out and only two checkout counters are open. Both are exactly the same. There are two people in front of you and they don't have a lot of groceries. The lines are moving quickly. The only difference is that one cashier seems annoyed and isn't interacting with their customers while the other cashier is smiling and appears to be engaging. Which line do you want to be in? I want to be in line with the happy cashier as opposed to the grouchy one. The same thing goes for you as a caregiver.

If you seem annoyed, expressionless, or standoffish, patients aren't going to feel comfortable or safe with you. Residents have confided in me about other aides, not in a gossiping kind of way, but out of real concern. I had a patient tell me that whenever a certain CNA worked with him, every time he asked the aide to take him to the bathroom, the woman would roll her eyes, sigh heavily, slam the door, bang furniture around, and shake her head. All these things are unacceptable. Going to the bathroom is a basic human need we are all entitled to. And I can't imagine anything more difficult than having to ask someone to assist you in going to the bathroom. You may feel annoyed with residents at times, but you have to do your best not to show it. My grandmother has vowed never to return to a nursing home because of the cruelty that she experienced there by an employee who clearly did not want to care for her. In her case, it was abuse, and our family reported the staff member. It only takes one bad experience that will stay with a person, and their family members, for the rest of their lives.

Don't be that "bad experience."

Be the reason that someone is smiling and grateful to have you in their lives.

"Kindness is a passport that opens doors and fashions friends. It softens hearts and molds relationships that can last lifetimes."

JOSEPH B. WIRTHLIN

REAL-LIFE EXPERIENCE

Think back to a time when you were sick. I'm not talking about a cold, but when you were really ill. The kind that lands you in the hospital when you don't want to be there. Last December, I found myself in the hospital with a kidney infection. It was so severe that I almost lost one of my kidneys, and I was in my late twenties. The entire experience was terrifying and surreal. For years I had been in the position of caring for people who were sick, so to be on the flip side of that was difficult for me. In a single day, I went from being a happy, healthy, independent woman to a distraught, dependent, and disabled person. It was terrifying on so many different levels, and I'll never forget it. The reason I won't ever forget it is because of how I was treated when I was there. The majority of the staff there were excellent, extremely kind, knowledgeable, and efficient, but there were some who were not so great. Those healthcare workers are the ones whom I'll always remember. I remember being bent over in wrenching pain, ugly crying, feeling as though I was about to throw up, lying on an uncomfortable bed while a nurse stood over me, telling me in an annoyed tone to stop moving so much. All while she pulled on my arm and stuck me with an IV needle. In my most vulnerable state, what I needed was kindness and understanding besides medication, and I received rudeness and impatience. Again, don't be that person.

PRACTICAL TIPS ON HOW TO HAVE A FRIENDLY DEMEANOR

Treat Others Well.

My mother taught me as a little girl to treat others the same way that I want to be treated, regardless of a person's race, economic status, nationality, age, religion, disability, gender, job, or political affiliation. Today I'm a grown woman, and I hold this practice with me still. On days where I'm feeling tired or run down, I don't let my exhaustion or frustration get the best of me. I remember what my mother taught me. I know what it's like to be treated poorly, and it doesn't feel good, so I try my best not to treat others like that.

Being Positive Improves Your Health.

Studies have shown that when you're sick, being positive, or having people who are positive around, improves your health. Think about it. Do you want individuals who are always happy and upbeat around you or individuals who are always depressed and miserable? I like the saying, "You become the five people with whom you hang around with." Think about this too: Do you like the five people with whom you hang out with? Do they bring joy to your life in different ways? Or do they bring drama and negativity, constantly ruining the good moments and good life you're trying to build for yourself? It's essential to have a positive mindset and to surround yourself with positive people. You won't know it until you try it, but trust me, it will relieve your stress! It will make you feel good about life. So on your days off, make it a priority to do something fun. Think outside the box! Having fun doesn't have to cost you anything. I once had a picnic by myself in the backyard. I laid out a blanket, ate lunch, and listened to a podcast. That, to me, was fun and relaxing. Another time, I met a friend at a national park. We walked, had great conversations, and took in the fresh air and beautiful scenery around us. We had an amazing time, and it was fulfilling. At the end of this chapter, you'll have a chance to make a list of five relaxing yet fun activities that you can do on your days off that will bring you the small doses of joy you need to stay positive and healthy. Chores don't count, by the way!

Smile!

For goodness sake, it's not going to hurt you, and I promise you're not going to overstretch your *zygomaticus major* muscle (that's the muscle that lets you smile). Some people act as though it will, but I promise you it won't. When you smile, it makes you more approachable to others. Smiling is contagious, in a very good way. Do you know how many people have told me that I'm the only one who smiles when I enter their room? That blows my mind. Are there that many unhappy and distressed people in the world? Yes. And how sad. And we all could choose to be one of them. But even on days when I'm having a bad day, I smile because it automatically puts me in a better mood. Well, that and ice cream, but that's a completely different topic. Spread kindness throughout your day, not sadness. All it takes is a smile. And even if you fake it, it still works and makes people smile! (They may smile because you look kinda funny doing it, but that doesn't matter.) There are very few free things in our power that we can do that can make someone else feel good and appreciated. A smile is one of them.

Random Acts of Kindness

These are spur of the moment things you can do that will make you and someone else feel great. A few examples are:

- Bring your patients a glass of water or a snack if their diet allows for it

- When you're on your way to the kitchen or the breakroom, ask whoever is near you, or your shift coworker, if you can get them anything while you're there

- Leave the good parking spot for someone else who might need it more, or to surprise someone who might feel "Hey, today is my lucky day!" Because the good parking spot is finally available for them

- Compliment yourself. This is a hard one for me, but it's gotten easier over time. I focus on one physical attribute I have, and then all throughout the day, I lift myself up with positive thoughts and words. For example, I look at myself in the mirror and say, "Nina, you have beautiful eyes." I know this sounds weird, but trust me, it's worth it. If you don't love yourself, with flaws and all, who else is going to?

HELPFUL RESOURCES

"The 5 Most Intriguing Benefits Of Friendliness In The Workplace" article by Heather Harper

"How Do Negative & Positive Attitudes Affect the Workplace" article by Lisa McQuerrey

"BENEFITS OF A POSITIVE ATTITUDE: HEAL YOUR MIND AND BODY" article by Health Conscious

The Power of Kindness: The Unexpected Benefits of Leading a Compassionate Life book by Piero Ferrucci

"The Power of Kindness" YouTube video, by Simon Sinek

PERSONAL COMMITMENT

These are the three things I commit to working on
to have a more friendly demeanor:

1. _____

2. _____

3. _____

These are five relaxing and fun things that I'm going to do next time I have some time off. I commit to doing at least one per day off, and what matters is that they're fun TO ME:

1. _____

2. _____

3. _____

4. _____

5. _____

Date:_____ My Signature: _____

INTENTIONAL CAREGIVING

ACKNOWLEDGMENTS

The following individuals have been part of my journey from a young woman to an entrepreneur:

My extraordinary Mommy bear, Lisa Miles. Your unconditional love and support mean so much to me. You are the woman I aspire to become. I love you more than words can describe!

My phenomenal business mentor Gary Seibert (sbrassociation.com), thank you for your mentorship, patience, and for believing in me even when I didn't believe in myself.

My exceptional friend Heather Anderson (Kadesh.biz) you have been a terrific business and spiritual mentor. Thank you for your guidance, humility, and grace you have shown me throughout the years.

My incredible editor Linda Ruggeri (theinsightfuleditor.com), thank you for your kindness, patience, knowledge-sharing, and professionalism throughout my book-writing journey. I would have never been able to write this book without you!

My remarkable father, Dennis Cooper, thank you for your unwavering love, guidance, and prayer for me over the years. You have been a consistent male figure in my life and I'm proud to be your daughter.

My amazing grandparents Grace and Jerry Beard, I'm thankful for your unfailing love, the abundance of wisdom, and countless laughs throughout the years. You've been the best ice cream buddies a granddaughter could ever ask for!

My dearest Rebecca Lewis (IG planet_bexx) you have always been there for me through the good times and the not so good times. Thank you for the many years of laughter, joy, consistency, and sisterhood. You are the best bosom friend a woman could have ever asked for!

ABOUT THE AUTHOR

CHRISTINA MILES

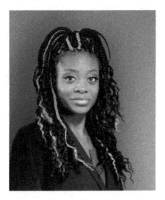

Christina Miles is an experienced certified nursing assistant who lives in Southeast Pennsylvania with her rambunctious dog Lucy. When she isn't busy caring for her patients, she enjoys traveling around the world, meeting people from all walks of life, listening to podcasts, going to business conferences, watching documentaries, and writing. She is passionate about improving the patient care system and working conditions for caregiving professionals. Her motto in life is to "Always treat people with kindness" and "Eat more ice cream."

Leave a Review

If you enjoyed this book, please consider leaving a review on Amazon.com or Goodreads.com so other readers may discover it too.

Connect with Christina

For comments and suggestions please write to
caregiveracademy1@gmail.com.

Follow Christina and her projects on
LinkedIn and Instagram.

CPSIA information can be obtained
at www.ICGtesting.com
Printed in the USA
BVHW040139150521
607049BV00005BA/870

9 780999 278093